Preeclampsia

Edited by Hassan Abduljabbar

Published in London, United Kingdom

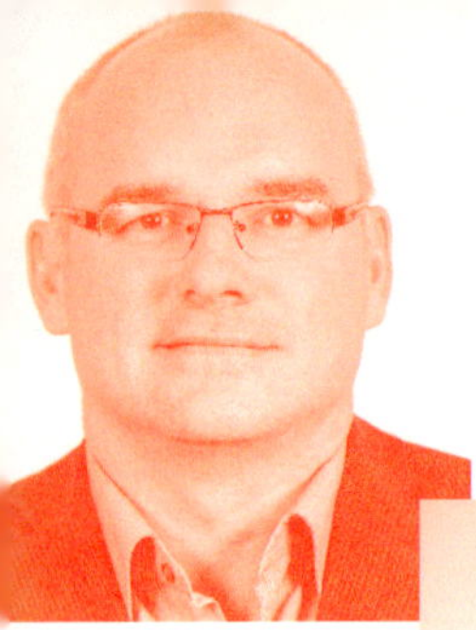
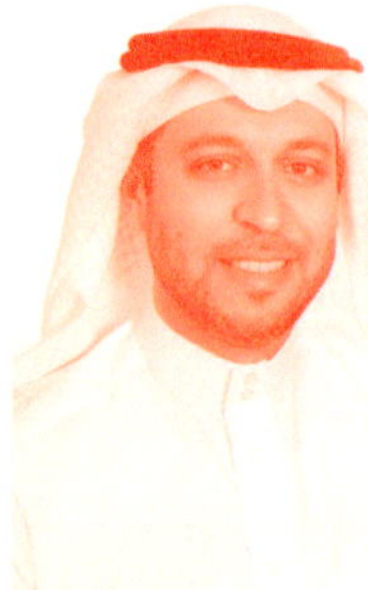
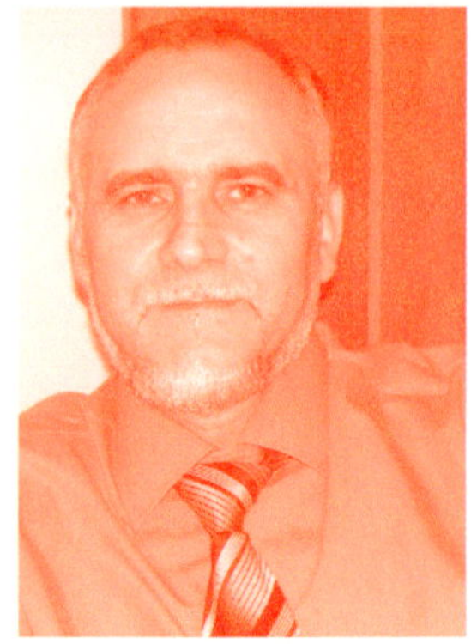
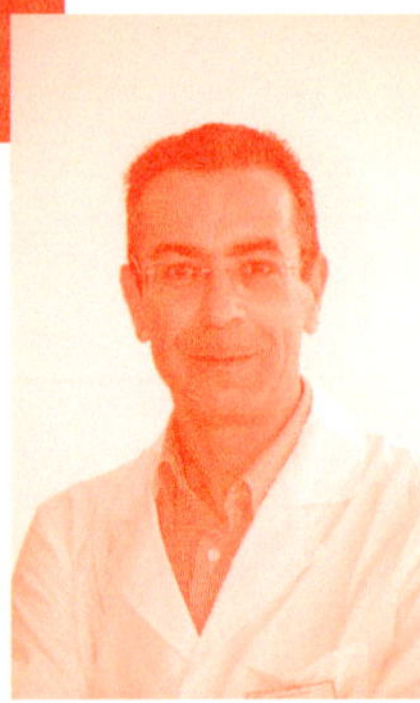
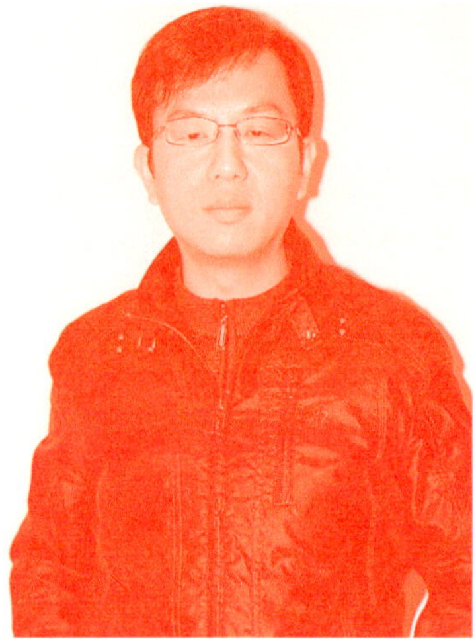
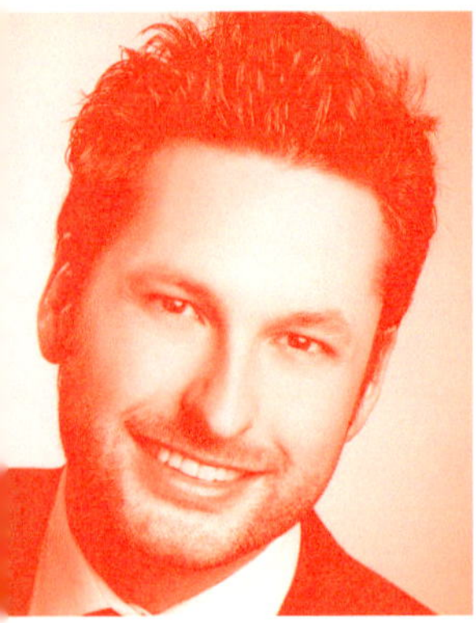
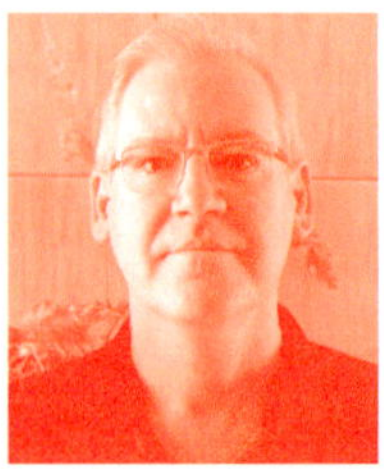

IntechOpen

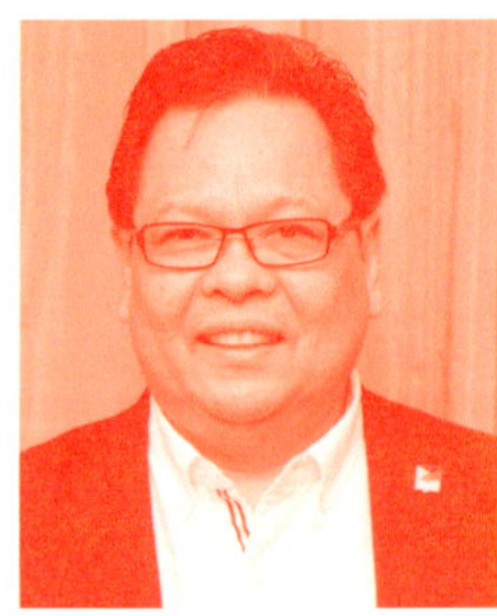
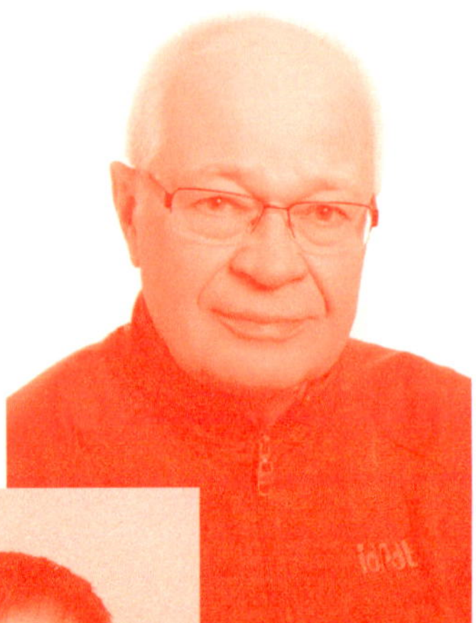
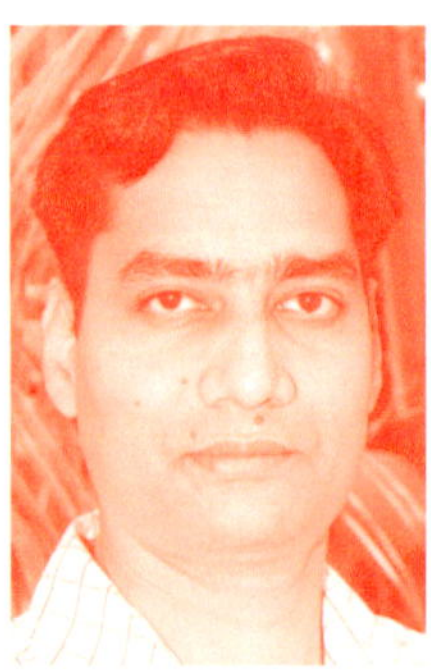
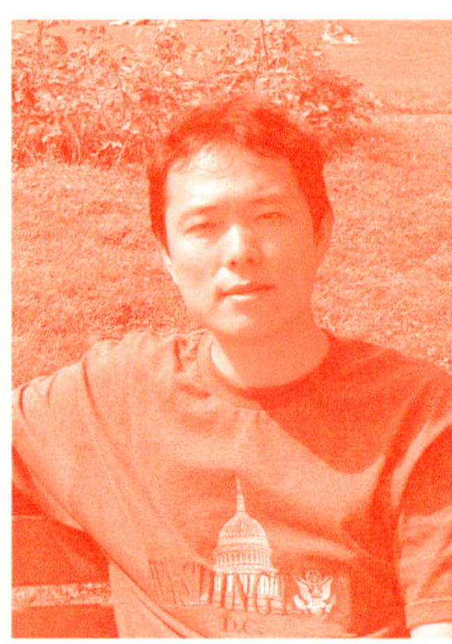
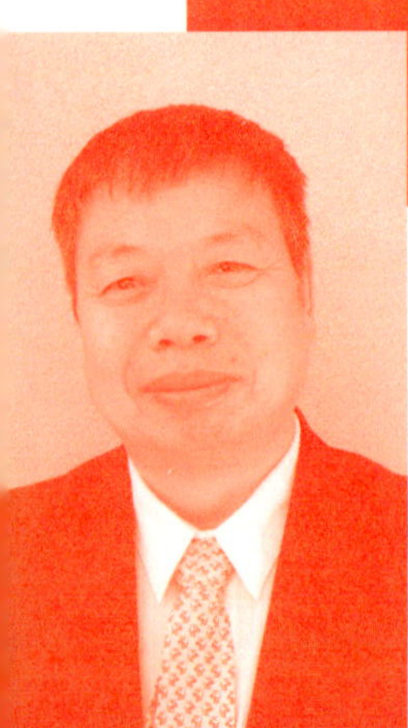
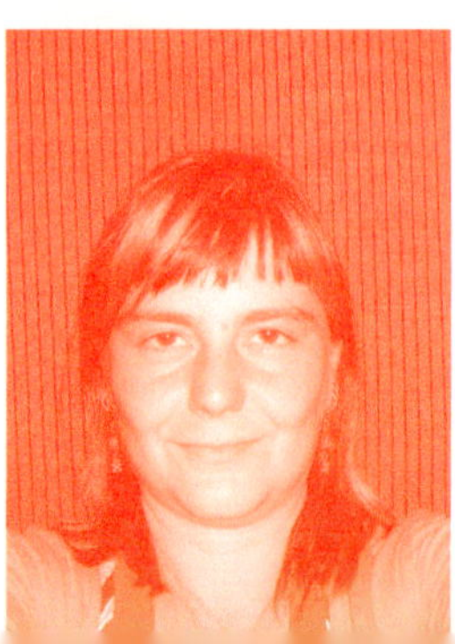

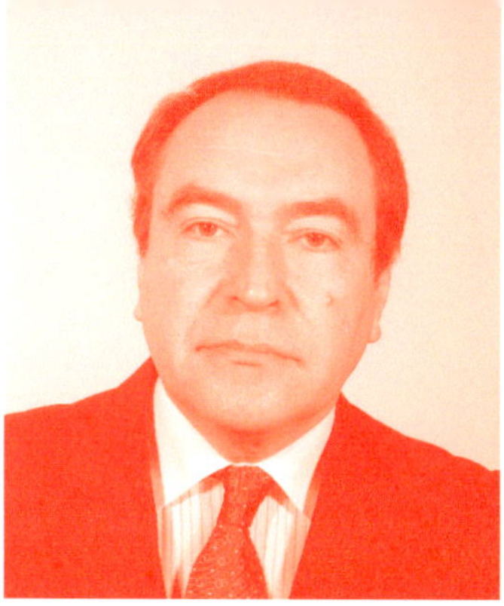
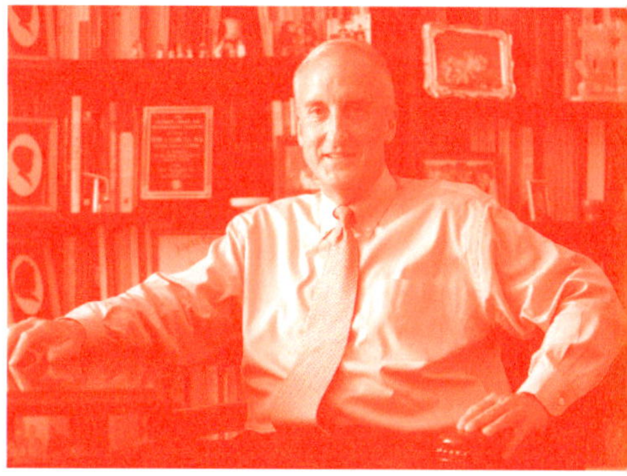
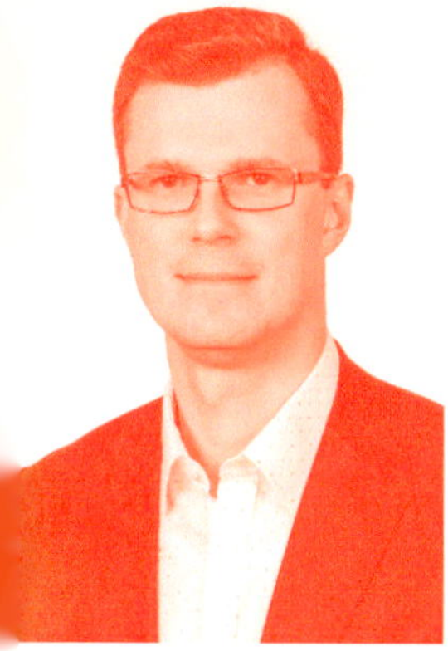
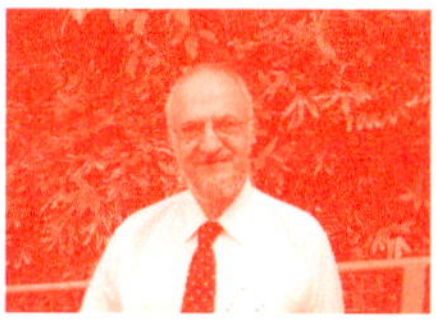
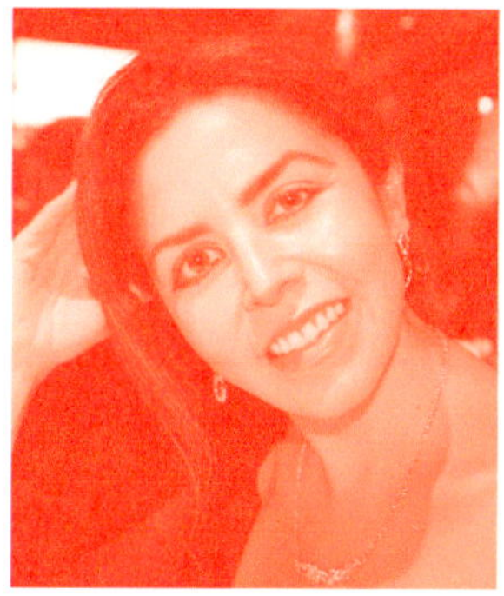

Supporting open minds since 2005

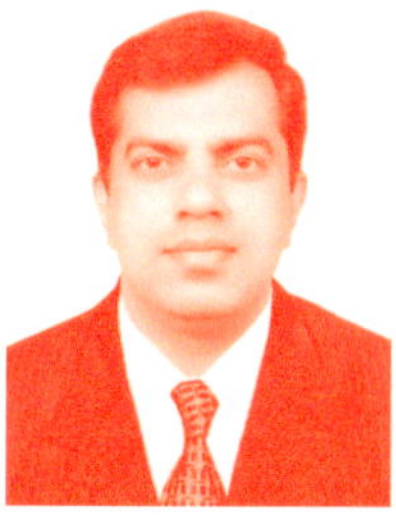
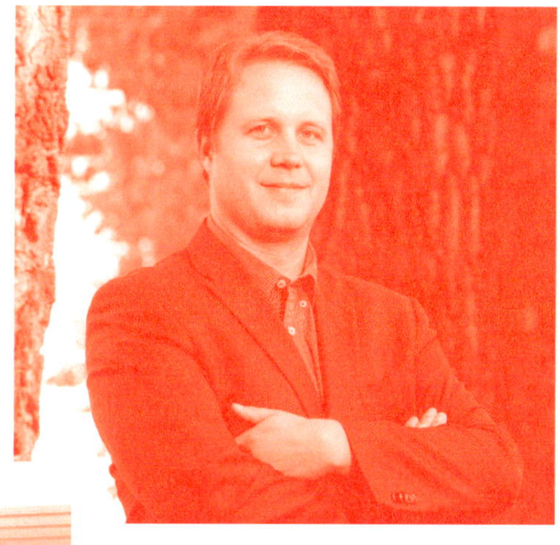
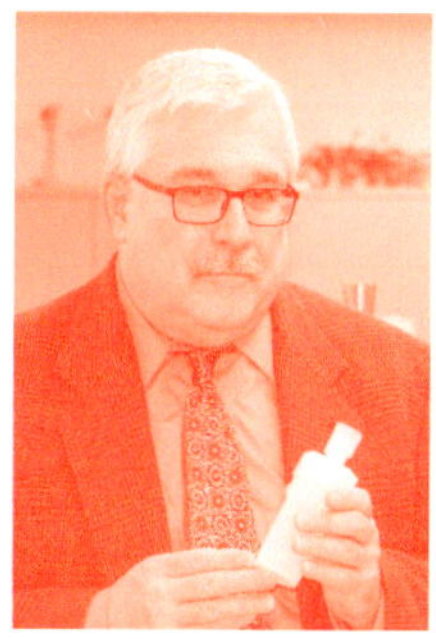
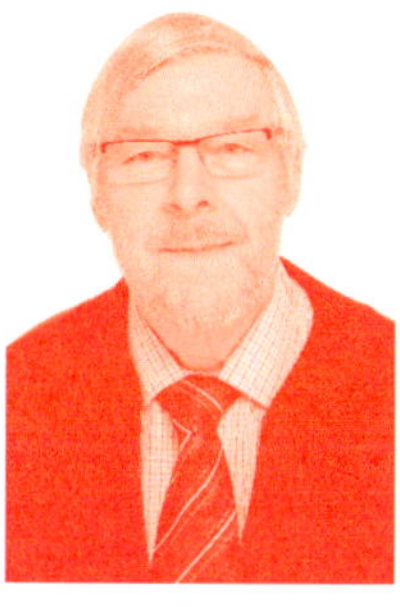
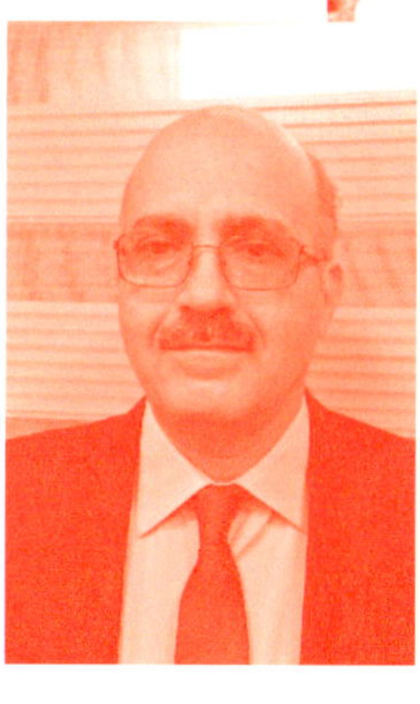
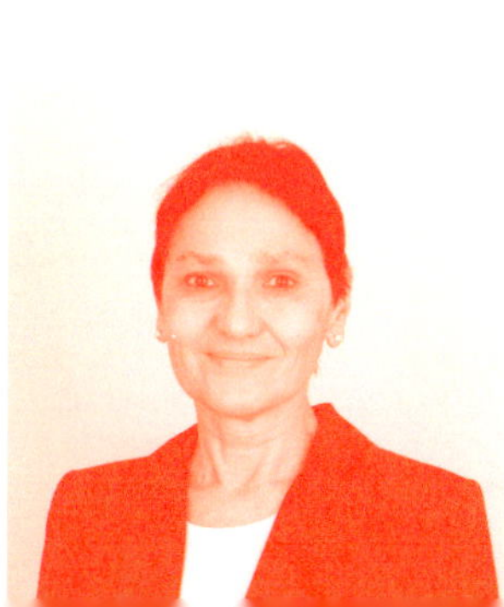
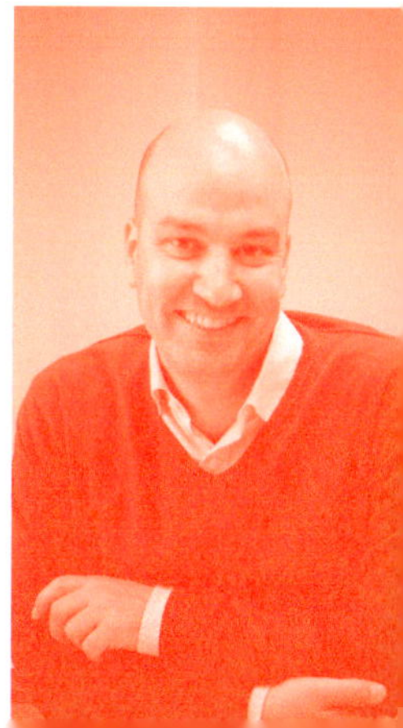

Preeclampsia
http://dx.doi.org/10.5772/intechopen.94691
Edited by Hassan Abduljabbar

Contributors
Simmi Kharb, Nissar Shaikh, Seema Nahid, Firdous Ummunnisa, Asma Gul, A. Al Basha, W. Yahia, F. Al Hail, H. Elfil, E. Abdulla, MM Nainthramveetil, Mahammad Zubair, S. Khan, N. Korichi, S. Alkhawaga, H. Ismail, S. Yaqoob, Fred Chasalow, Ivan Cavar, Antonio Sesar, Anita Pusic Sesar, Katarina Cvitkovic, Dmytro Konkov, George Belkaniya, Victor Rud, Levon Dilenyan, Larisa Klimas, Alina Piskun, Liana Puchalska, Hemamalini Vedagiri, Premkumar Kumpati, Ajithkumar Balakrishnan, Janaranjani Murugesan, M.A Imraan, Mashael Abdulrahman M.S. Al Khelaifi

First published in London, United Kingdom, 2022 by IntechOpen
IntechOpen is the global imprint of INTECHOPEN LIMITED, registered in England and Wales, registration number: 11086078, 5 Princes Gate Court, London, SW7 2QJ, United Kingdom
Printed in Croatia

British Library Cataloguing-in-Publication Data
A catalogue record for this book is available from the British Library

Additional hard and PDF copies can be obtained from orders@intechopen.com

Preeclampsia
Edited by Hassan Abduljabbar
p. cm.
Print ISBN 978-1-83969-294-9
Online ISBN 978-1-83969-295-6
eBook (PDF) ISBN 978-1-83969-296-3

For EU product safety concerns:
IN TECH d.o.o., Prolaz Marije Krucifikse Kozulić 3, 51000 Rijeka, Croatia, info@intechopen.com or visit our website at intechopen.com.

Meet the editor

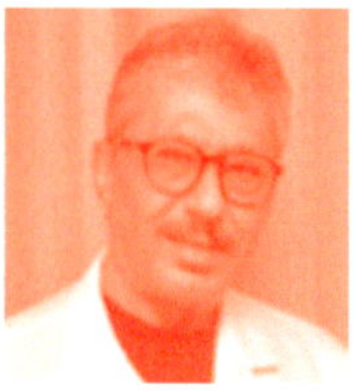

Hassan S. Abduljabbar, MD, FRCSC, American Board Diplomate, is a professor at the College of Medicine, King Abdulaziz University, Saudi Arabia. He is also the president of the Saudi Society of Obstetrics and Gynecology and the Federation of Arab Gynecology Obstetric Societies (FAGOS). He is a referee for many international scientific journals. He is also an examiner for graduate degrees as well as for the Saudi and Arab board exams. Dr. Abduljabbar has published more than fifty articles and edited three books.

Contents

Preface

Preeclampsia is one of the most common complications of pregnancy. It is characterized by high blood pressure and organ damage, most often of the liver and kidneys. Severe cases may cause hemolysis, low platelets and impaired liver function, kidney dysfunction, pulmonary edema, shortness of breath, and visual disturbances. Preeclampsia usually occurs in the third trimester but can occur as early as 20 weeks.

Preeclampsia/eclampsia is one of the three leading causes of maternal morbidity and mortality worldwide. During the past 50 years, there has been a significant reduction in the rates of eclampsia, maternal mortality, and maternal morbidity in developed countries.

This book includes six chapters. Chapter 1 discusses pathophysiology of preeclampsia, Chapter 2 describes how vitamin D deficiency can be a factor in developing preeclampsia, Chapter 3 deals with cellular changes that occur with preeclampsia, Chapter 4 describes how preeclampsia can lead to organ dysfunction, Chapter 5 explores the gestational endotheliopathy that may lead to complications, and finally, Chapter 6 examines ophthalmic complications of preeclampsia.

Hassan Abduljabbar
Dr. Erfan & Bagedo General Hospital,
Obstetrics and Gynecology Department,
Jeddah Fertility Center,
Jeddah, K.S.A.

Section 1

Pathophysiology

Chapter 1

Role of Spiral Steroids in Pregnancy and Pre-Eclampsia

Fred Chasalow

Abstract

My laboratory discovered a new type of steroids. The structure of these steroids is unique in three ways: (i) they have 23, 24 or 25 carbon atoms – no other known vertebrate steroid has more than 21 carbon atoms; (ii) they are phosphodiesters – no other steroid phosphodiesters are known; and (iii) some of them have a spiral steroid at carbon 17 – no other endogenous spiral steroids are known. In total, our laboratory had elucidated the structure and path of biosynthesis for more than 20 related compounds. We have developed an LC–MS method and a MS–MS method to measure the compounds in small samples (< 1 ml). Synthetic compounds with similar spiral steroids (e.g., spironolactone) function as potassium sparing hormones but there were no known endogenous hormones with this function. We propose that the natural spiral steroids have that function. Endogenous compounds with these functions would have important roles in the physiology of pregnancy, pre-eclampsia, and eclampsia. This chapter will review the proposed physiology and pathology of the spiral steroids during pregnancy. There are many details to confirm but this is a useful paradigm.

Keywords: hypertension, proteinuria, hypokalemia, edema, spiral steroids, Ionotropin

1. Introduction

Here is a brief history of the milestones on the discovery path that led to the discovery of phosphodiester spiral steroids and the recognition of their function as potassium sparing hormones (KSH):

- In the 1950s, Szent-Gyorgyi proposed that digoxin was not a drug but was an analog of a natural hormone [1].

- In the 1970s, Walsh and others developed RIAs for digoxin [2].

- In the 1980s, Graves observed that, during the third trimester, patients with pre-eclampsia had unknown materials in their serum that cross-reacted in his assay for digoxin [3].

- Chasalow observed that patients with Smith-Lemli-Opitz Syndrome (SLO) were K+ wasting, had high levels of two polar steroids, of which one was a Digoxin Like Material (DLM). By two weeks of age, both compounds were undetectable. In normal infants there were four polar steroids, three of which were DLM and all four were not detectable by 2 weeks of age. We proposed that SLO was an enzyme defect in a previously unknown pathway that produced a compound that was potassium sparing [4].

- Bradlow observed that some human breast fluids had high K+ levels [5]. Chasalow and Bradlow speculated that the high K+ levels were caused by a DLM the SLO patients did not make. This started a collaboration to identify the DLM [6].

- In the 1990s, Hamlyn claimed to have isolated 13 μg of 'ouabain' from 80 liters of human plasma and proposed that it was the DLM hormone anticipated by Szent-Gyorgyi [7]. Hamlyn has not been able to confirm that the material he isolated was present in serum samples from a patient with pre-eclampsia by any method other than by RIA. If it were ouabain that he isolated, the concentration in serum that he reported would have little or no consequences [8]. The chemical properties of his material differed from the unknown DLM we found in newborn serum and in human breast cyst fluids [6, 8].

- In the 2000s, based on the identical assay for digoxin, Chasalow isolated six novel steroids from animal and human serum [9].

- In the 2010s, Chasalow identified the structures of the first 6 steroids and proposed a pathway for biosynthesis with the added atoms derived from malonyl-CoA [10]. Three of the compounds are phosphodiester conjugates of spiral steroids. The other 3 are potential precursors. Later, we corrected the biosynthetic pathway [11].

- In the 2020s, we observed that as early as 22 weeks of gestational age, precursors of spiral steroids were elevated in serum from women with pre-eclampsia but were not elevated in serum from normotensive women of similar gestational age. We confirmed by MS–MS spectrometry that these were steroid phosphodiesters, like those present in newborn serum and human breast cyst fluids [12].

- Precursors were elevated in 11 of 19 women with pre-eclampsia and in only 1 of 20 normotensive pregnant women. No other proposed marker correlates with more than 35% of affected women [13]. We propose that this divides patients with pre-eclampsia syndrome into two diseases. This would be a major advance in developing treatment protocols [14].

In summary, this chapter proposes a new paradigm to account for the symptoms of pre-eclampsia. The paradigm also accounts for the long-term increased risk of both cardiovascular disease and end-stage renal disease in affected women and their offspring [15, 16].

2. Biochemistry of steroid phosphodiesters

This section describes the biochemistry of steroid phosphodiesters. I have used Ionotropin as a key word in every paper about steroid phosphodiesters. I suggest other investigators do likewise.

Ionotropin was the name we assigned to the steroid phosphodiester that was present in human serum and not present in serum from infants with SLO syndrome.

We now know that there are two compounds that fit the definition of Ionotropin – C339 and C341. C339 and C341 are both present in human blood and were not present in serum from an infant with SLO. This usage would be equivalent to using glucocorticoid as a hormone type name and cortisol and corticosterone as specific compounds.

2.1 Symbol convention

Based on the steroid fragment observed on mass spectroscopy, we assigned a symbol with four characters in the 'Zabc' format [11]. The Z identifies which phosphodiester is present in the molecule: (a) C = phosphocholine, (b) P = phosphoethanolamine and (c) X = unknown. The 'abc' identifies the mass of the steroid fragment observed in a positive ion mass spectrum. The method is not antibody dependent. Anyone with a mass spectrometer can identify the appropriate symbol for any steroid phosphodiester. Note that, potentially, there could be isomers that share the same mass ion and phosphodiester fragment.

C339, C341, E339, and E341 were all present in bovine adrenal extracts but neither E339 nor E341 were detectable in serum from any species that we tested. This observation points to adrenal cortex as the site of synthesis.

2.2 Numbering convention

When only phosphodiester steroids with 23 carbon atoms were known, it did not make much difference which carbon was designated # 22 or # 23. Both are part of the E-ring. However, when we recognized that the added carbon atoms were derived from acyl-CoEnzyme A, we have revised the numbering scheme to reflect their common origin (**Figure 1**).

2.3 Mass spectrometric methods

Two basic methods were used. The first method used LC–MS with Atmospheric Pressure Chemical Ionization (APCI) in the positive ion mode [9]. Voltages were

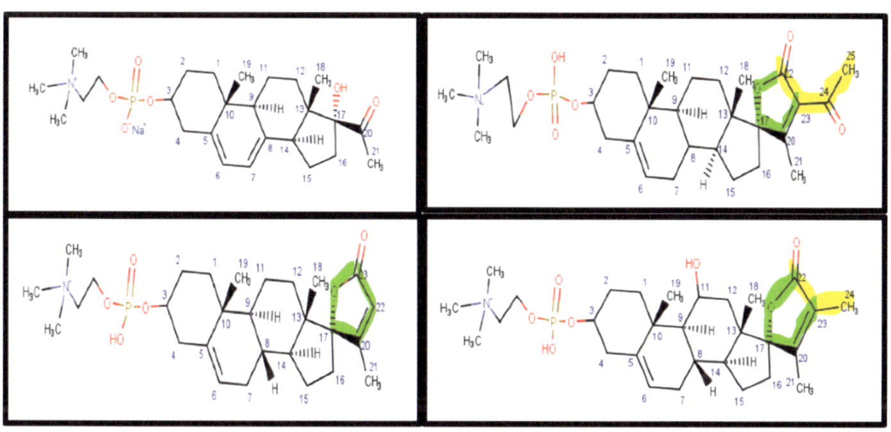

Figure 1.
Structures of representative steroid phosphodiesters. Starting in the upper left and going counter-clockwise, the compounds are C313, C339, C351, and C381. Carbon 17 is the spiral steroid. Ring E is painted green and the extra side-chain carbons are painted yellow. C339 is shown with the original, classical numbering scheme [17]. The revised scheme is shown for both C353 and C381. The new scheme recognizes carbon 22 as the carboxyl carbon of the CoEnzyme A acyl group. This numbering scheme clarifies the proposed common origin of the extra carbon atoms.

selected to minimize fragmentation. The second method used direct injection into a quadrupole ion trap mass spectrometer [12]. Spectra were collected both with and without an additional fragmentation voltage. MS–MS analysis was also used to confirm parent-fragment ion relationships.

Steroids have molecular masses in the range 270 to 400 Da. The smallest steroid fragment from a phosphodiester has a molecular mass of 297 Da and the largest fragment thus far identified has a mass of 413 Da.

2.4 Trial and error (T&E) determination of chemical composition

Table 1 illustrates the use of the T&E method to propose a composition for C381. As shown on Line 7, only one composition of carbon, hydrogen, and oxygen atoms can form a molecule with a mass of 398 Da - $C_{25}O_4H_{34}$. Readers are invited to test other molecular compositions to generate a molecule with a mass of 398 Da. Similar T&E tables have been used for each of the steroid fragments we identified. The observation that only one composition fits the mass may be a coincidence but it certainly was useful. Occam's razor suggests that the phosphodiesters are all related, as precursors and/or metabolites. If this is not true, then there must be other, as yet undetected, phosphodiester steroids.

Line	Carbons	Oxygen	C + O	H-maxHH H-Max	H-Req	m/z	Delta
1	23	5	356	48	42	398	3
2	23	6	372	48	26	398	11
3	24	4	352	50	46	398	2
4	24	5	368	50	30	398	10
5	24	6	384	50	14	398	18
6	25	3	348	52	50	398	1
7	**25**	**4**	**364**	**52**	**34**	**398**	**9**
8	25	5	380	52	18	398	17
9	26	2	344	54	54	398	0
10	26	3	360	54	38	398	8
11	26	4	376	54	22	398	16
12	27	2	356	56	42	398	7
13	27	3	372	56	26	398	15

Line: Each line describes a trial of a possible composition.
Carbons: The number of carbon atoms in this specific trial.
Oxygen: The number of oxygen atoms in this specific trial.
C + O: The contribution of the carbon and oxygen atoms to the mass.
Hmax: Maximum number of hydrogen atoms – 2+ 2 for each carbon atom.
Hreq: Difference between m/z and "C + O".
m/z: mass of the steroid fragment plus 17 Da- the fragment has lost an OH.
Delta: the number of delta necessary to complete a molecule. Delta is ½ the difference between Hmax and Hreq. Delta is the number of rings and double bonds in the molecule. The basic steroid structure has four rings. Ring E contributes 3 delta – ring, alkene, and the carboxylic acid. Thus, delta must be 7 or larger.
Conclusion: Line 7 (in bold) shows the molecular composition is $C_{25}O_4H_{34}$ and delta must be 9.
Isomers for the proposed structure of C381 are not eliminated by the T&E analysis. The same analysis has been done for each steroid fragment.

Table 1.
Trial and error (T&E) analysis of composition of C381.

2.5 Spiral steroid biosynthesis

All of the newly discovered compounds are either phosphocholine (PC) steroid diesters or phosphoethanolamine (PE) diesters. The presence of the choline phosphodiester was confirmed by ^{31}P-NMR (**Figure 2**) and by the presence of a characteristic fragment at m/z = 184 Da in mass spectra. In humans, both choline and ethanolamine may be essential nutriments. The phosphodiester could be added to a steroid by condensation with CDP-serine and subsequent decarboxylation (see **Figure 2**). Based on the phosphodiesters we have identified, the acceptor steroid seems to be 17α-hydroxy-pregna-5,7-dienolone. Shackleton has isolated this compound from patients with SLO [19] and Slominski has confirmed that enzymes exist to convert 7-dehydrocholesterol to the same precursor [20].

The working theory is that the extra carbons are added by condensation of C313 or E313 with an acyl CoA (**Figure 3**). The three most common CoA acyl groups are: (i) acetyl, (ii) propyl, and (iii) acetoacetyl. The three lead to steroids with 23, 24, and 25 carbon atoms, respectively (**Table 2**). The three carboxylic acid intermediates were identified by their mass spectra. We can identify compounds which have hydroxy groups by MS–MS fragmentation (by loss of 18 Da). However, it does not identify which specific carbon atom had been hydroxylated.

C341 is the major spiral lactone in adult serum with lessor quantities of C337 and C339. These compounds differ by stepwise reduction of the two alkenes in their common C313 precursor. For cholesterol biosynthesis, the Δ7–8 bond must be reduced first because cholesterol has a Δ5–6 alkene but not a Δ7–8 bond. The same enzyme could be responsible for the reduction of Δ7–8 alkene to reduce C337 to C339. A second reduction step is necessary to reduce the Δ5–6 bond. Although testosterone is reduced to form the 5α derivative, that enzyme substrate specificity requires a Δ4, 3-ketone. As the phosphodiester blocks the ketone at carbon-3, that enzyme could not reduce C339. There is a reductase that generates 5β-metabolites. It forms cholic acid for bile. Thus, an enzyme with this specificity would produce the 5β-C341 isomer. Note that digoxin is also a 5β steroid.

The takeaway lesson from **Figure 4** is that the 5β isomer would fit like a key into a specific binding site in which the 5α isomer would not fit. The stereo-specificity of C341 is probably significant because the major weak androgen in humans (but not in most other species) is DHEA-S, which is a 5α-steroid. If C341 were a 5α- steroid, then both DHEA and 5α-dihydrotestosterone could both interfere with its function by binding at the receptor for C341, whatever it might be. Recall that spironolactone also binds to both the androgen receptor and the KSH receptor. In fact, this cross-

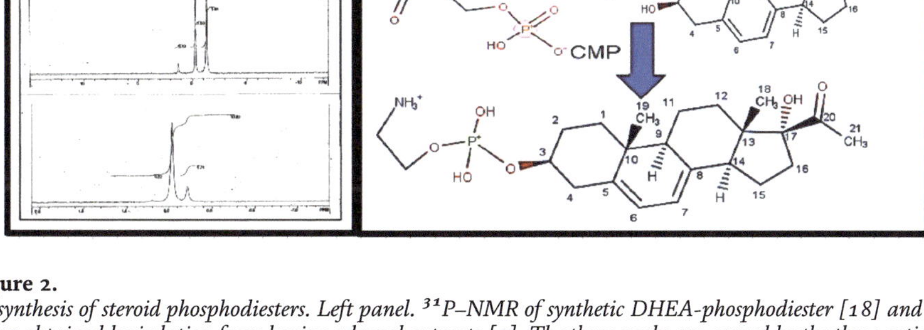

Figure 2.
Biosynthesis of steroid phosphodiesters. Left panel. ^{31}P–NMR of synthetic DHEA-phosphodiester [18] and of C341 obtained by isolation from bovine adrenal extracts [9]. The three peaks are caused by the three cations (H+, Na+, and K+). Right Panel. Condensation of serine-CDP with 17α-OH-pregna-5,7-dienolone [19, 20] to form E313. We do not know the order of the two reactions – Decarboxylation and esterification. Mass spectroscopy confirmed E313 was present in adrenal extracts [9].

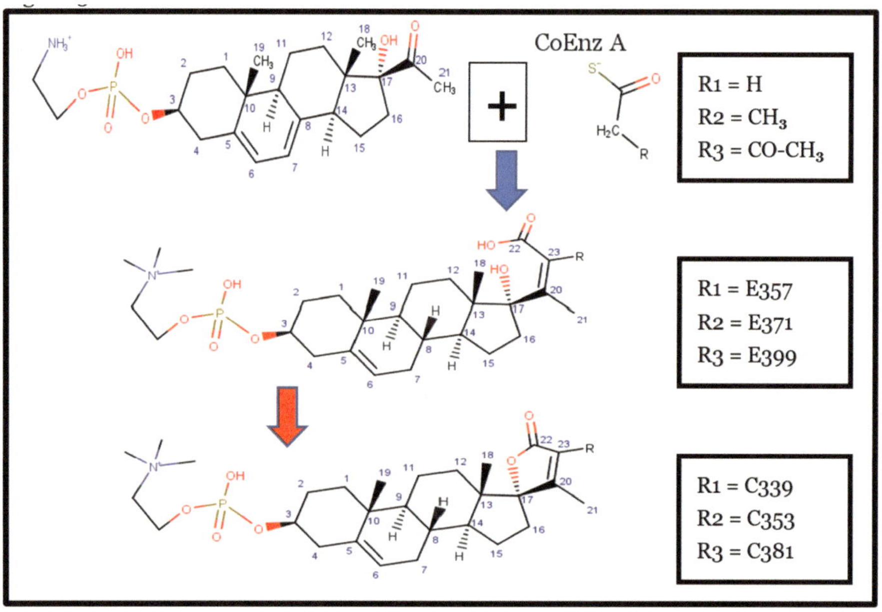

Figure 3.
Synthesis of phosphodiester spiral steroid lactones. Starting with E313, this figure shows the formation of the spiral steroid lactones. There are several steps at the Blue arrow: N-methylation, Δ7–8 reduction, and condensation with acyl-coenzyme A. The lactone ring formation occurs at the Red arrow. The order of the steps has not been positively determined. The three boxes show how the three Acyl groups lead to the three different side chains at carbon 23. The conversion of PE compounds to PC compounds (N-methylation) may occur at any step.

binding makes spironolactone a less desirable pharmaceutical. Chickens and turkeys do not use DHEA as a weak androgen. This may explain why their serum has C339, but not C341, as the major spiral lactone [21].

2.6 Tissue specificity

Question: why do we need all three classes of spiral lactones?

Answer: Tissue specificity. Pre-pubertal children only have 23-carbon lactones. Gonad extracts and serum from pregnant women have 24-carbon lactones. Milk and high K+ breast cysts have 25-carbon lactones. There are multiple forms of the NaK-ATPase. We need to isolate each of the forms and evaluate their binding constants to the different spiral steroids at the different forms of NaK-ATPase.

Question: why do need both PE and PC phosphodiesters?

Answer: Best answer at present is the PE compounds are for storage until needed. N-methylation is ACTH dependent. Thus, as part of the stress response the epinephrine increases glycolysis and the spiral lactone increases heart efficiency [10]. We suggest (without direct proof) that the same process occurs during childbirth.

2.7 Summary of biochemistry

The last discovery of a novel steroid was of aldosterone and that occurred in the 1950s. The general consensus has been that all of the steroids were already known. Hamlyn's claim to the discovery of endogenous ouabain has not been widely accepted [7]. They reported isolating 13 μg from 80 liters of plasma (0.2 ng/ml). Blaustein, one of his colleagues, has even published a paper asking, "Why is endogenous ouabain not more widely accepted?" [22]. Nicholls replied saying, "Ouabain, a circulating hormone secreted by the adrenals, is pivotal in cardiovascular disease,

Symbol	Alkenes	Composition	Other features
Steroids with 21 carbon atoms			
C313*@	Δ5; Δ7	C21O3H30	
C329*#@	Δ5; Δ7	C21O4H30	Hydroxy
Steroids with 23 carbon atoms (formed by condensation with Acetyl-CoA)			
C337*@	Δ5; Δ7; Δ20	C23O3H30	!
C339*@	Δ5; Δ20	C23O3H32	! Ionotropin
C341*@	Δ20; 5β	C23O3H34	! Ionotropin
C361*@+	Δ5	C23O4H36	22 - carboxyl
C363*@+	5β reduced	C23O4H38	22 - carboxyl
Steroids with 24 carbon atoms (formed by condensation with Propyl-CoA)			
C353	Δ5, Δ20, 23-CH3	C24O3H34	!
C369#@	Δ5, Δ20, 23-CH3	C24O4H34	! hydroxy
C371#@	5β, Δ20, 23-CH3	C24O4H36	! hydroxy
C389@+	Δ5, 23-CH3	C24O5H36	22 - carboxyl
Steroids with 25 carbon atoms (formed by condensation with Acetoacetyl-CoA)			
C381¶	Δ5, Δ20, 23-CO-CH3	C25O4H34	!
C413#&	Δ5, Δ20, 23-CO-CH3	C25O6H34	! di-hydroxy

**Compounds purified to near homogeneity.*
@ Mass spectrum also identified phosphoethanolamine (Exxx).
! Spiral steroid lactone.
 # Site of hydroxy unconfirmed. Likely possible sites are at carbons 11 & 16. Compounds with an extra hydroxy fragment by loss of water (18 Da). This eliminates hydroxy groups at the axial carbons –18, 19, and 21.
+Carboxyl compounds must be protonated in the positive ion spectrum.
¶ This fragment was detected in milk extracts from cows, sheep and goats.
& This fragment was only detected in fetal calf serum extracts.

Table 2.
Steroid phosphodiesters identified by Mass Spectroscopy.

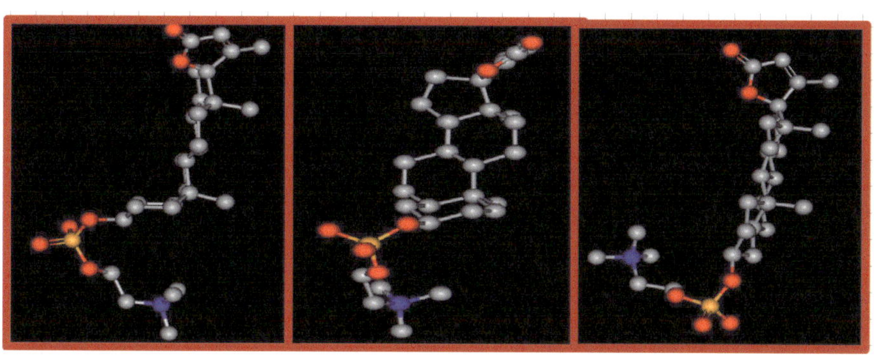

Figure 4.
3D images of C341, a spiral steroid. Color code: carbon – grey; oxygen - red; phosphorus – orange; nitrogen – blue. Hydrogen atoms are not shown in these images. From bottom to the top, the ring designations are A, B, C, D, & E. Panel A and B show two different views of the 5β stereoisomer of C341. Ring A and Ring E, the spiral ring, are both perpendicular to the plane generated by Rings B, C and D. Panel C shows the 5α stereoisomer. Note that in the 5α stereoisomer, Ring A, B, C, and D are co-planar and only the plane of Ring E is perpendicular to the plane of the four rings. In both stereoisomers, the PC fragment has free rotation around the steroid plane.

fact or fantasy?" [23]. Nicholls described two criteria required for an endogenous hormone: [a] biosynthetic pathway and [b] a method of assay not dependent on antibody specificity. Endogenous ouabain satisfies neither criteria. In fact, Baecher developed an ultrasensitive LC–MS method to measure serum levels of "endogenous ouabain" down to less than 2 pg./ml and could find none [24]. This section describes both a biosynthetic path to the spiral steroids and methods to measure spiral lactones by mass spectroscopy. It is unclear what Hamlyn measured but it is time to consider the role of the spiral lactones as the real endogenous KSH.

3. Physiology of spiral steroid phosphodiesters

This section describes our knowledge of the function of spiral steroids. As spiral steroid phosphodiesters are also present in oysters, the function is not limited to mammals but is probably common throughout the animal kingdom [25]. Plants seem to use cardiotonic glycosides for the same function. Amphibians use marinobufagenin and related compounds as poisons to discourage predators [26]. We have not measured spiral steroids in amphibian serum to identify which spiral steroid is used in their internal physiology. Note that marinobufagenin can only be obtained from amphibian skin after extensive hydrolysis. As such, it would not be expected to be present in serum.

3.1 Why do we need to regulate intracellular K+

For creatures living in the sea, ocean electrolytes are 460 mM Na + and 10 mM K+. This ratio closely resembles the electrolyte ratio in plasma 145 mM Na + and 4 mM K+. In contrast, intracellular electrolytes are 10 mM Na + and 140 mM K+. Although we know about the role of mineralocorticoids to recover needed Na+, until 2016, there were no known mechanisms to maintain intracellular K+ levels or to recover K+ in the kidney.

Most plants and animals have high levels of both Na + and K+ in their tissues and/or fluids. Thus, there is little need for a concentration mechanism for life forms that have free access to environmental foodstuffs. However, *in utero*, fetuses only have access to maternal serum electrolytes via the placenta. The fetus must concentrate K+ about 20-fold and must maintain the intracellular levels, despite passive diffusion of K+ from a high K+ intracellular fluid to a low K+ extracellular fluid.

3.2 Background to endogenous K+ sparing hormones or diuretics

None known.

3.3 Background to synthetic K+ sparing diuretics (KSD)

There are two types of chemicals classified as KSD and they function by different mechanisms. The Steroid-type, represented by spironolactone, activates K+ transport by the NaK-ATPase. The AT type, represented by amiloride or triamterene, interfere with passage of Na + ions through the epithelial sodium channel (ENaC). This reduces the need to 'pump' Na + out of cells [27].

Steroid-type KSDs include: digoxin, ouabain, spironolactone, eplerenone, marinobufagenin. Common features include:

- E-ring lactone with 5, 6, or 7 atoms

- Binding to most digoxin specific antibodies
- Inhibition of NaK-ATPase in the usual assay
- Pressor activity in vivo

Spiral steroid phosphodiesters have all four features.

AT Type compounds function by interfering with Na + passage through ENaC. This activity reduces the diffusion of Na + from high Na + extracellular fluids to low Na + intracellular fluids. This leads to lower intracellular osmotic pressure and 'spares' intracellular K+. The net affect is to generate a positive inotropic response [27].

3.4 Potassium accumulation in human breast cyst fluids

Earlier, because breast cysts were suspected of being precursors for breast cancer, the biochemistry of the cysts was investigated [5]. Based on electrolyte composition, there were two types. Type 1 had high K+ levels (60–100 mM) and Type 2 had potassium electrolyte levels resembling normal serum (~5 mM). We investigated DLM levels in cyst fluid samples obtained in the normal course of patient care [6]. DLM was only present in the Type 1, high K+, samples and the levels were 10 times the levels detected in serum from normal women or men. We proposed that the basis for the high K+ levels was the presence of a K+ regulating hormone. Type 1 fluids were used to develop methods for extraction and chromatography. The new methods were different from that used to isolate 'ouabain' or 'digoxin' from plasma [7]. Doping experiments confirmed that the new method would not extract authentic cardiotonic glycosides. However, we could not collect sufficient Type 1 cyst fluid to purify the steroid phosphodiesters. In retrospect, it seems likely that C381 was the spiral steroid actually present in the Type 1 fluids.

4. Biochemistry and physiology of spiral steroids during pregnancy

Spiral steroids function as endogenous KSH and regulate both intracellular K+ levels and K+ recovery [27]. Regulation of K+ is particularly important during pregnancy because the fetus receives all of its nutrition via the placenta and does not have access to K+ rich foods (**Figure** 5).

4.1 Fertilization

After ova are fertilized, the cells divide and multiply. The growing cells need K+ for their intracellular fluids. We detected C369 and E369 in bovine ovarian extracts. C369 is a spiral steroid with 24 carbon atoms and a hydroxy group at an unidentified location (**Figure 6**). I propose that C369 is the spiral lactone that functions as KSH for fertilized ova. Both C329 and C353 are present in serum from pregnant women. C369 was present in serum from 10 out of 10 (5 males and 5 females) obligate heterozygotes for SLO [29]. At present, there is no explanation for the presence of C369 in serum from the heterozygotes but not in other men or women.

4.2 Maternal spiral steroids during second trimester

At 22–24 weeks of gestational age, there are five steroid phosphodiesters in maternal serum: C313, C329, C341, C353 and C381 (**Figure** 7). C313 and C329 have

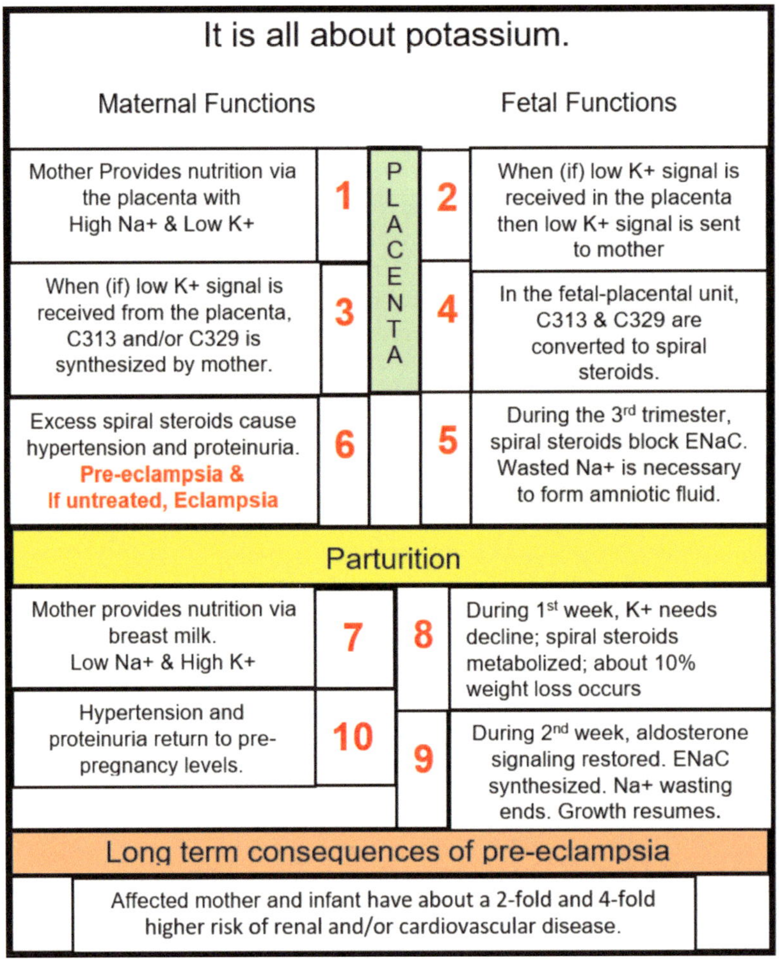

Figure 5.
Schematic regulation of potassium during pregnancy. The figure shows the proposed relationship between potassium and spiral steroids during pregnancy. Most of the processes are known, but the significance of the steroid phosphodiesters had not been recognized [28].

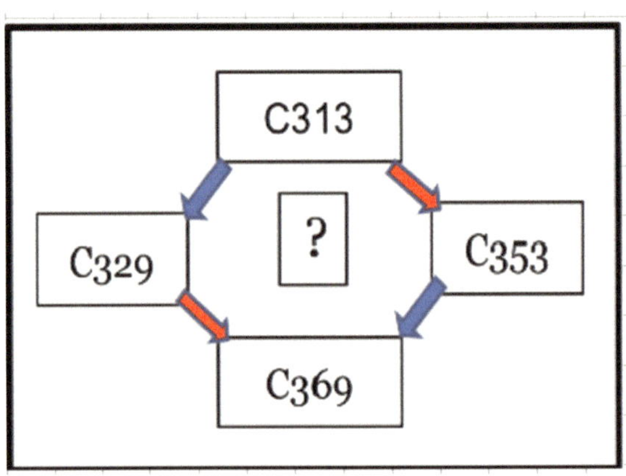

Figure 6.
Biosynthesis of C369. Red Arrows: condensation with Propyl-CoEnz A; Blue Arrows: Hydroxylation at unconfirmed carbon atom. C353 and C369 are both spiral steroids.

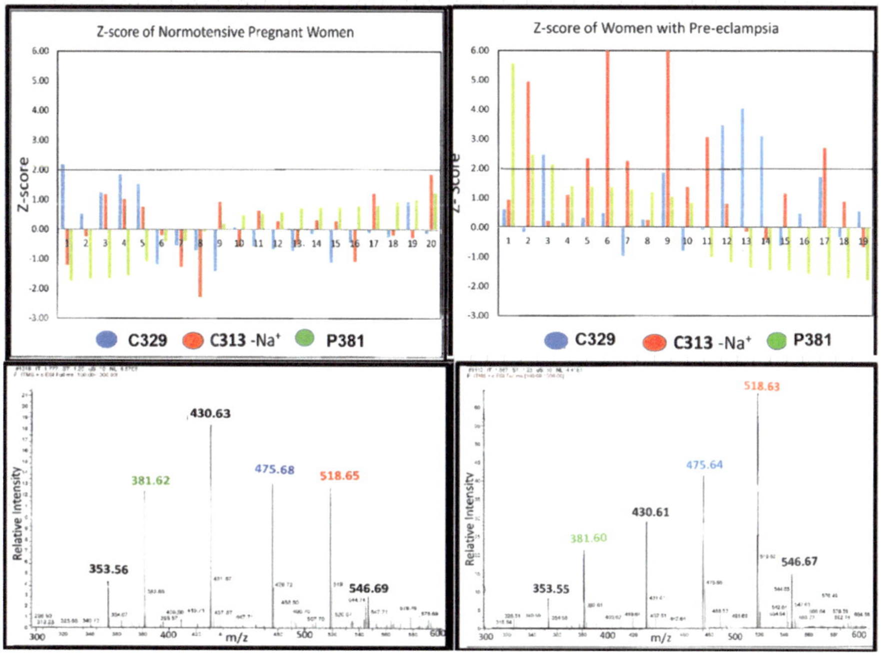

Figure 7.
Steroid phosphodiesters during the second trimester. Serum samples (22–24 weeks of gestational age, n = 20 normotensive women; n = 20 women with pre-eclampsia) were obtained from Global Alliance for the Prevention of Prematurity and Stillbirth (GAPPS). Left column: normotensive women; Right column: women with pre-eclampsia. Top: Z-scores based on intensity of miltefosine as internal control. Bottom: Representative mass spectra. Method of analysis: For each spectrum, the intensity of each ion was compared to the intensity of the ion generated by miltefosine (hexadecyl-phosphocholine). The mean and standard deviations of ions from the normotensive women were calculated and used to generate Z-scores for each of the 40 samples. The Z-scores for each sample were graphed as a cluster [12]. Ions are identified in ***Table*** *3.*

21 carbon atoms. The other three are spiral steroids with 23, 24, and 25 carbon atoms, respectively.

4.3 Aldosterone signaling changes in the 3rd trimester

During the third trimester, there is a so-called 'aldosterone-signaling defect.'

In fact, there are actually two distinct aldosterone-signaling *changes* during pregnancy and these do not resolve until 2 weeks post-natal [30].

One change reduces the activity of the ENaC. This is equivalent to an AT type activity of KSD. This leads to Na + wasting in the fetal kidney and is a key, necessary step in producing the electrolytes for the amniotic fluid.

The second change is equivalent to the S Type of KSD, leading to increased activity of the NaK-ATPase pump. The increase leads to increased intracellular K+ in the fetal and maternal heart. The K-Ca- exchange mechanism increases calcium levels in the heart and results in a calcium-dependent, increased pressor response in both the fetal and maternal compartments.

The increased fetal pressor response is necessary because, as the fetus grows, the arterial resistance increases due to the increased length of the arterial bed. The increase in the maternal pressor response is needed because of the increased size of the vascular bed in the placenta. For both processes, the biology was known but the relationship to endogenous KSH was unknown because the existence of a KSH was unrecognized.

In summary, the aldosterone signaling changes are not a defect but are normal changes that are necessary during the second and third trimester.

4.4 Preparation for milk production

Milk is unique in that it is the only major extracellular fluid with K+ levels higher than Na + levels – 12-17 mM of K+ vs. 5–6 mM Na+ [31]. A KSH function should be necessary to concentrate K+ from plasma (4–6 mM) to the higher K+ levels in milk. In fact, milks from goats, cattle and sheep all had high levels of C381, suggesting that it is the KSH required to accumulate high levels of K+. This observation suggests that the NaK-ATPase isoform in breast tissue may be specific for C381, rather than for any other spiral lactone.

4.5 Post-natal

Post-natal, infants are fed milk, which is high in K+, and the need for a KSH ends but serum levels of spiral steroids remain detectable for about two weeks. Infants remain Na + wasting and usually lose about 10% of their birth weight. By two weeks of age, the need for KSH is over; the spiral steroids have been metabolized; aldosterone function is restored; Na + wasting ends; growth resumes [30]. Mother and infant "live happily ever after."

4.6 Summary of the role of spiral steroids during pregnancy

Spiral steroids, acting as KSHs, play a key role in K+ regulation during pregnancy. Ionotropin with 23 carbon atoms is the primary KSH for maternal function. The 24 carbon atom compounds, C353 and C369, function in the gonads and in the fetal-placental compartment. As the mother prepares for milk production, C381, the spiral steroid with 25 carbon atoms, directs the accumulation of K+. Ionotropin (C339 and/or C341) and C381 are DLM. C353 and C369 have the same spiral lactone epitope and are probably DLM, but we have not confirmed that suggestion by isolation and testing of extracts. All of these compounds are phosphocholine steroid diesters. The corresponding phosphoethanolamine steroid diesters are present in extracts from tissues that ordinarily synthesize steroid hormones but are only present in trace amounts (if at all) in serum [9].

m/z (Da)	Symbol	Color	# of C	Origin of ion	Comment
353*	C353	Black	24	Fragment	Spiral steroid
381*	C381	Green	25	Fragment	Spiral steroid
475!	C329	Blue	21	Loss of TMA	Precursor
518	C313	Red	21	Na + ion	Precursor
546	C341	Black	23	Na + ion	Spiral steroid

The identify of each steroid ion was confirmed by MS–MS analysis. All parent ions were Na + ions. C313 is the precursor for C341; C329 is the precursor for C369. One of the precursors was elevated in 11 of 19 samples from women with pre-eclampsia.
** The ion detected is the steroid fragment after loss of the phosphocholine.*
! The ion detected is derived from Na + ion after loss of trimethylamine (TMA).

Table 3.
*Identification of phosphodiester steroids in serum (**Figure 7**).*

5. Physiology of spiral steroids in pre-eclampsia

Pre-eclampsia is a syndrome, not a disease [32]. As a syndrome, the diagnosis is made by hypertension and proteinuria. The symptoms can begin as early as 20 weeks of gestation [33–35]. For many patients with pre-eclampsia, there is little consequence during pregnancy. Monitoring and bed rest are often recommended. However, about 6–10% of affected women develop life-threatening hypertension and/or seizures. The only treatment is immediate C-section [15]. After C-section, the seizures and hypertension usually resolve.

In addition to the classical symptoms, during the third trimester, many affected patients also develop hypokalemia [36, 37]. In fact, there is a statistically significant ($P < 0.05$) inverse relationship between maternal serum K+ levels and maternal blood pressure [35]. Publications from 3rd world countries describe hypokalemia in patients with pre-eclampsia but publications from 1st world countries do not recognize hypokalemia as a symptom or risk factor.

There are several things to note in **Figure 7**.

- At 22–24 weeks of gestation, serum DLM is undetectable by most assays [38].

- Although C353 (an ion at m/z = 353 Da) and C341 (an ion at m/z = 546 Da) were detected by mass spectroscopy, both ions were of low intensity and might not be detected in a DLM assay. The variability of the intensities for these two ions did not correlate with disease status.

- Neither C381 (detected at m/z = 381 Da) nor C329 (detected at m/z = 475 Da) were detected in outdated human plasma [9].

- For both C313 (detected at m/z = 518 Da and C329 (detected at m/z = 475 Da) there was a significant increase ($P < 0.05$) in mean serum levels6in women with pre-eclampsia and many samples had Z-scores greater than 2.0.

We used three different statistical methods to evaluate the ion intensity of the C313, precursor of Ionotropin. First, we compared the mean and standard deviation of the of the samples from the normotensive women with the corresponding data from the women with pre-eclampsia. Second, we used Rank sum analysis. This method does not assume a normal distribution and is considered more robust than methods that imply a normal distribution. Third, we used the mean and standard deviation of the normotensive women to show Z-scores for all 40 samples. This set of data is presented in the clusters in **Figure 7**. There were 12 samples from the women with pre-eclampsia with Z-scores over 2 for either C313 or C329; there was only one sample from a normotensive woman with Z-score over 2. This distribution is statistically significant at the $P < 0.01$ level. With all three methods, the differences are statistically significant at the $P < 0.05$ level. Although there was an increase in the concentration of precursors, DLM was undetectable at this stage of gestation [39].

This data portends converting pre-eclampsia from a syndrome to at least two diseases. One disease, Type A, characterized by elevated levels of at least one of the spiral steroid precursors (either C313 or C329), a second disease, Type B, characterized by normal levels of the precursors. The takeaway lesson from this study is hypertension and proteinuria seem to be symptoms of more than one disease [40].

5.1 Proposed biopathology of pre-eclampsia

- Inadequate implantation leads to inadequate fetal K+.
- To compensate, the placenta secretes excess spiral steroid precursors – either C313 or C329.
- Mother responds by converting the spiral steroids to C341 or C369.
- C369 acts as a KSH in the fetal-placental unit, which further depletes maternal K+.
- Fetal hypokalemia prevents normal growth. This may be the process that leads to low birthweight infants.
- Hyperspirolemia (high serum levels of C341 or other spiral steroid phosphodiester) functions as an KSH and leads to maternal hypertension and proteinuria. Hyperspirolemia would be detected as a DLM.
- Continuous hyperspirolemia would lead to life-threatening seizures.
- Sustained hyperspirolemia damages heart and kidney and increases life-long disease risk (**Figure 8**).

The initial underlying biopathology seems to be inadequate placental implantation [41, 42]. Investigators have measured many, many hormones as possible risk factor or mediators, but none predict more than 35% of the patients who develop the symptoms, none predict hypokalemia, none predict risk of life-threatening hypertension [43–45], and none provide a biochemical basis for the increased life-long risk of renal or cardiac disease.

5.2 Significance of changes in aldosterone signaling

If fetal K+ levels were inadequate, the placenta should synthesize spiral steroid precursors, C313 and C329 [12]. This leads to their increase in the maternal circulation. In turn, these compounds are converted to spiral steroids which function as KSHs. Elevated KSH has been documented in patients with pre-eclampsia as increased DLM levels. This seems to be a normal third trimester process occurring during the second trimester. The preeclampsia symptoms would be caused by interference in function of the ENaC in the kidney and by increased pressor activity in the heart due to the secondary increase in Ca++.

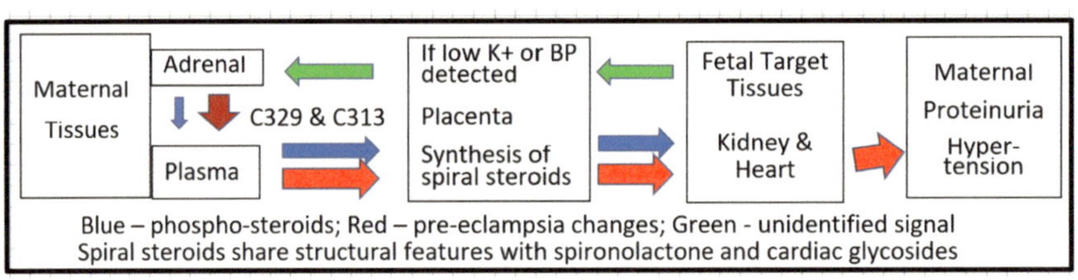

Figure 8.
Changes in spiral steroids during pre-eclampsia. This figure integrates the regulatory process with the normal role of spiral steroids acting as KSH. The biology has been known. The underlying biochemistry was unknown prior to the discovery of the spiral steroids. The shuttling back and forth of steroid phosphodiesters between the mother and the fetal-placenta unit is similar to the synthesis and function of estriol.

5.3 Pilot study results

C313, the precursor for C341, was detected in serum from pregnant women by the ion at m/z = 518 Da (generated by {a} 313 Da from the steroid fragment, {b} + 183 Da from the PC fragment, {c} + 23 Da from the Na+, and {d} -1 Da from the loss of the H+ = 518 Da.). 7 of 20 women diagnosed with preeclampsia had elevated levels (Z > 2) of C313 in serum collected at 22–24 weeks of gestation. Just like overdose of KSDs, elevated levels of C341 in maternal serum would be expected to lead to maternal hypertension, proteinuria and hypokalemia.

C329, the precursor for C369, was detected in serum from pregnant women by the ion at m/z = 475 Da. This ion is generated by loss of trimethyl amine (59 Da) from the Na + ion at m/z = 534 Da. 4 of 20 women diagnosed with preeclampsia had elevated levels (Z > 2) of C329. There was a statistically significant increase in concentration of C329 in the affected patients when compared to the normotensive control group. This would be expected to lead to increased levels of a KSD in the fetal circulation without corresponding increases in the maternal circulation. However, the incidence of samples with Z > 2 for C329 did not reach statistical significance; a larger sample size will be needed.

C329 is the precursor of C369. C369 was not detected in pre-pubertal children but was present in 10 of 10 obligate heterozygotes for SLO. There is no report of increased incidence of maternal hypertension or proteinuria in this group. Three of the 40 samples had high levels of C369, presumably associated with heterozygote carrier status for SLO.

A third group, 9 of 20 women with preeclampsia, had normal levels of both C313 and C329 at 22–24 weeks of gestation. There may be three different patterns: [a] high levels of C313 leading to maternal hypokalemia and life-threatening hypertension, [b] high levels of C329 leading to self-treatment of the fetal hypokalemia without generating maternal life-threatening hypertension, and [c] a 3rd group of patients with an unrelated origin of their symptoms. Overall, only about 5–10% of women with pre-eclampsia develop seizures and/or life-threatening hypertension later in pregnancy. The existence of 3 diseases sharing symptoms of proteinuria and hypertension might be the explanation for the lack of progress in developing therapy for these syndromes.

5.4 Post-partum

The green bars and peaks in **Figure 7** show the C381 levels in serum from pregnant women. At 22–24 weeks of gestation, only one of the 40 samples had elevated levels of C381, characterized by a score of Z > 2. There was no significant difference between the serum levels of C381 of normotensive pregnant women when compared to the serum levels of C381 from women with pre-eclampsia. C381 could stimulate milk production without affecting maternal heart or kidney function.

If during gestation, the mother had pre-eclampsia, long-term damage may have occurred due to persistent hyperspirolemia. Animal models treated with plant-derived cardiotonic steroids develop long-term heart and kidney consequences [46, 47].

6. Therapy for pre-eclampsia

6.1 Failed therapies

6.1.1 Phosphodiesterase inhibitors

One hypotheses is pre-eclampsia can be treated with phosphodiesterase inhibitors, including sildenafil citrate [48, 49]. However, Podymow writes, “As currently understood, the hypertension of preeclampsia is secondary to placental under perfusion, thus lowering systemic BP is not believed to reverse the primary pathogenic process." [50].

6.1.2 Digibind

Digibind is an FAB isolated from an antibody to digoxin and is used to treat patients with hypertension caused by digoxin toxicity [51]. As there are elevated levels of DLM in serum from women with pre-eclampsia, Digibind has been tested to determine if it would reduce hypertension in women with preeclampsia [51]. Infusion with Digibind does lead to a prompt decrease in blood pressure in affected women. However, the effect is short lived. Within 12 hours, blood pressure has returned to pre-therapeutic levels. The interpretation was that ane unknown agent was bound to the FAB and excreted. However, additional amounts were synthesized, leading to continued hypertension. The effort, if any, to confirm the identity of the unknown agent has not been published.

6.1.3 Monoclonal antibodies to Marinobufagenin

Marinobufagenin is a poison originally isolated from toad skin extracts [52]. Abi-Ghanem, with polyclonal antibodies, developed a chemifluorescent immunoassay [53]. Agunanne used the assay to confirm elevated marinbufagenin levels in women with preeclampsia [54]. Fedorova developed monoclonal antibodies and observed there was an unknown factor in serum of Dahl rats that was detected by their monoclonal antibody [55]. In the first publication, it was characterized as marinobufagenin-like, then as endogenous marinobufagenin [56]; most recently, just as marinobufagenin [52]. However, there are no publications describing characterization of marinobufagenin, or any plausible precursor or metabolite, from any mammalian source, other than by immunoassay.

Despite not knowing the true identity of the 'factor' detected by these antibodies, investigators have proposed a role for marinobufagenin in pre-eclampsia in women [57]. I do not doubt that there is at least one unknown substance that cross-reacts with marinobufagenin-specific antibodies in serum from patients with pre-eclampsia. I doubt that it is marinobufagenin.

6.2 Proposed therapy

The Pilot Study showed increased levels of one of the spiral steroid precursors, C313 or C329, in the maternal circulation. The corresponding spiral steroids are C341 and C369. High levels of C369 were present in obligate heterozygotes with SLO but these women do not have pre-eclampsia [29]. Thus, the cause of hypertension and proteinuria would seem to be C341. This leads to two significant therapeutic suggestions: [1] monitor disease progression with C313 and [2] treat with C369 or its precursor, C329. The goal would be to stimulate KSH activity in the fetus without stimulating the function of a KSH in the maternal circulation.

6.3 Proposed diagnostic method

The pilot study was designed to maximize the chance of a clear positive response. In fact, statistically that was achieved. However, it is likely that the elevated level of C313 did not appear suddenly at 22 weeks of gestation. A large study is needed to determine when the elevated precursor levels begin and, later in gestation, which spiral steroids are elevated in the patients who develop eclampsia or HELPP syndrome [15].

7. Conclusion

One general theme in endocrinology is, "One disease to a customer." If all symptoms experienced by a patient are not explained by the proposed biochemistry, the patient has a syndrome, not a disease. This chapter title tells the story, "It's all about potassium." None of the reviews that I found recognize the significance of hypokalemia as part of the disease.

In detail, several facts stand out: [a] there is little evidence that pre-eclampsia is a single disease, [b] the common characterization of pre-eclampsia as a syndrome does not include hypokalemia, [c] without considering the role of spiral steroids, there is no recognized mechanism that shows how inadequate placental implantation leads to all of the classical symptoms of pre-eclampsia, hypokalemia or to the long-term increased risk of coronary or renal disease.

Acknowledgements

I specifically wish to recognize three very special colleagues: Dr. Ron Bochner, Dr. H. Leon Bradlow and Dr. Sandra Blethen (Chasalow).

Colleagues included, Dr. Kathryn King, LIJMC, Dr. Sharon Nachman, LIJMC, Dr. Gary Jarvis, VA Medical Center, San Francisco, CA and by Dr. Constance John, VA Medical Center, San Francisco, CA. Dr. John encouraged me and made laboratory space and equipment available. My two laboratory chiefs were Michael Davis and Lori Pierce-Cohen. Dr. Forbes Porter and Dr. Christopher Wassif of the NICHD provided serum samples from patients and obligate heterozygotes with Smith-Lemli-Opitz syndrome. Dr. Alisha Romano provided serum samples collected in the normal course of patient care.

Marvin Applets were used for drawing, displaying and characterizing chemical structures and reactions, Product Version 21.1 ChemAxon (https://www.Chemaxon.com).

Funding statement

This research did not receive any specific grant from funding agencies in the public, commercial or not-for-profit sectors. Dr. Ron Bochner personally funded the pilot study of women with pre-eclampsia. The Smith-Lemli-Opitz Foundation funded the investigation of the patients with SLO syndrome. AMUR Research Corp funded most of the original investigations. Kerix funded the purification of the compounds with 23 carbon atoms and the investigation of the chemical formulas. This work was partially supported by the Research Service of the United States Department of Veterans Affairs. Current support from IOMA LLC.

Conflict of interest

The authors declare no conflict of interest.

Author details

Fred Chasalow

1 IOMA LLC, Belmont, CA, USA

2 VAMC, San Francisco, CA, USA

*Address all correspondence to: fchasalow@gmail.com

References

[1] Szent-Gyorgyi A. (1955) Chemical physiology of contraction in body and heart muscle. Academic Press. New York, NY. As cited in Labella FS. (1985) Endogenous digitalis-like factors: Introductory Remarks. Fed Proc. 44: 2780-2781.

[2] Walsh P, Crawford F, and Hawker CD. (1977) Measurement of digoxin by radioimmunoassay. Annals of Clinical and Laboratory Science. 7: 79-87.

[3] Graves S. (1987) The Possible role of Digitalislike Factors in Pregnancy-Induced Hypertension. Hypertension 10 {suppl I}: I-84-6.

[4] Chasalow F, Blethen S, and Taysi K. (1985). Possible abnormalities of steroid secretion in children with Smith-Lemli-Opitz syndrome and their parents. Steroids. 46: 827-843.

[5] Bradlow H, Fleisher M, Breed C, and Chasalow F. (1990). Biochemical classification of patients with gross cystic breast disease. N Y Acad Sci. 586: 12-16.

[6] Chasalow FI and Bradlow HL. (1990) Digoxin-like materials in human breast cyst fluids. Ann N Y Acad Sci. 586: 107-116. DOI:10.1111/j.1749-6632.1990.tb17797.x. PubMed PMID: 2162647.

[7] Hamlyn J, Blaustein M, Bova S, DuCharme D, Harris D, Mandel F, Mathews W, and Ludens J. (1991) Identification and characterization of an ouabain-like compound from human plasma. Proc Natl Acad Sci. 88: 6259-6263.

[8] Chasalow F, and Blethen S. (1990) Characterization of digoxin-like material in human cord serum. Ann N Y Acad Sci. 591: 212-221. PMID: 2142872.

[9] Chasalow F and Pierce-Cohen L. (2018) Ionotropin is the mammalian digoxin-like material (DLM). It is a phosphocholine ester of a steroid with 23 carbon atoms. Steroids 136:63-75. DOI:10.1016/j.steroids.2018.03.001. Epub 2018 Mar

[10] Chasalow F. (2018) A new concept: Ionotropin May Be a Factor in Mobilization for [a] the Flight or Fight response and [b] Childbirth. EC Paediatrics. 7: 909-918. DOI:10.31080/ecpe.2018.07.00341

[11] Chasalow, F. Phosphocholine Steroid Conjugates: Are these Compounds the Mammalian Cardiotonic Steroids? *Preprints* 2020, 2020070211. DOI:10.20944/preprints202007.0211.v1.

[12] Chasalow F, John C, and Bochner R. (2019) Spiral steroids as potential markers for pre-eclampsia: a pilot study. Steroids. Nov. 151: 108466. DOI: 10.1016/j.steroids.2019.108466. Epub 2019 Jul 26. PubMed PMID: 31351941

[13] Wu P, van den Berg C, Alfirevic Z, O'Brien S, Rothlisberger M, Baker P, Kenny L, Kublickiene K, and Duvekot J. (2015) Early Pregnancy Biomarkers in Pre-Eclampsia: A Systematic Review and Meta-Analysis. International Journal of Molecular Sciences. 16: 23035-23056. DOI:10.3390/ijms160923035.

[14] Leslie K, Thilaganathan B, & Papageorghiou A. (2011) Best Practice and Research Clinical Obstetrics and Gynaecology. Early prediction and prevention of pre-eclampsia. 25: 343-354. DOI:10.1016/j.bpobgyn.2011.01.002.

[15] https://pre-eclampsia.org/long-term-impact-healthcare-providers. Dated July 17, 2020

[16] Vikse B, Irgens L, Leivestad T, Skjaerven R, and Iversen B. (2008)

Preeclampsia and the Risk of End-Stage Renal Disease. N Engl J Med. 359:800-809. DOI:10.1056/NEJMoa0706790

[17] Nomenclature of Organic Chemistry: IUPAC Recommendations and Preferred Names 2013 (BlueE Book). Cambridge: The Royal Society of Chemistry (2014): 822.

[18] Chasalow F. (2000) Synthesis of DHEA-PC. Phospholipid drug derivatives. US Patent 6,127,349.

[19] Shackleton C, Roitman, E, Guo LW, Wilson WK, and Porter FD. (2002) Identification of 7(8) and 8(9) unsaturated adrenal steroid metabolites produced by patients with 7-dehydrosterol-delta-7-reductase deficiency (Smith-Lemli-Opitz Syndrome). J Steroid Biochem Mol Biol. 82: 225-32. Pubmed/12477489

[20] Slominski A, Zmijewski M, Semak I, Sweatman T, Janjetovic Z, Li W, and Zjawiony J. (2008) Sequential metabolism of 7-dehydrocholesterol to steroid 5,7-dienes in adrenal glands and its biological implication in the skin. PLoS ONE 4(2): e4309. DOI:10.1371/journal.pone.0004309.

[21] Chasalow F. (2019). Spiral Phosphocholine Steroids and DLM in Chicken Eggs (Gallus domesticus). EC Paediatrics 8: 01-12. DOI:10.31080/ecpe.2019.08.00593.

[22] Blaustein M. (2014) Why isn't endogenous ouabain more widely accepted? Am J Physiol Heart Circ Physiology. 307(5): H635-H639. DOI: 10.1152/ajpeart.00402.2014

[23] Nicholls MG, Lewis LK, Yandle TG, Lord G, McKinnon W, and Hilton PJ. (2009). Ouabain, a circulating hormone secreted by the adrenals, is pivotal in cardiovascular disease. Fact or fantasy? J Hypertens. 27(1): 3-8. DOI:10.1097/HJH.0b013e32831101d1.

[24] Baecher S, Kroiss M, Fassnacht M, and Vogeser M. (2014) Noendogenous ouabain is detectable in human plasma by ultrasensitive UPLC-MS/MS. Clin Chim Acta, 431: 87-89.

[25] Chasalow F. (2020). Phosphocholine Steroid Esters in Pacific Oysters (Crassostrea gigas). EC Pediatrics 9: 115-126. DOI:10.31080/ecpe.2020.09.00844.

[26] Tomaschitz A, Piecha G, Ritz E, Meinitzer A, Haas J, Pieske B, Wiecek A, Rus-Machan J, Toplak H, Marz W, Verheyen N, Gaksch M, Amrein K, Kraigher-Krainer E, Fahrleitner-Pammer A, and Pilz S. (2015). Marinobufagenin in essential hypertension and primary aldosteronism: A cardiotonic steroid with clinical and diagnostic implications. Clin Exp Hypertens, 37: 108-115.

[27] Kennedy R, Berlin J, Ng Y, Akera T, Brody T. (1986). Amiloride: Effects on Myocardial Force of Contraction, sodium pump and Na+/Ca++ Exchange. J Mol Cell Cardiol. 18: 177-188.

[28] Chasalow F. (2021). Pre-eclampsia: It's all about Potassium. In: Eclampsia. Ed. By Sharon Wright. Nova Science Publishers. Inc. New York. 63-113. ISBN: 978-1-53619-574-3

[29] Chasalow F, Blethen S. (2020). Steroid Metabolic Consequences of 7-Dehydrosterol Reductase Deficiency (SLO). EC Paediatrics 9.6: 60-69. DOI: 10.31080/ecpe.2020.09.00720

[30] Bizzarri C, Pedicelli S, Cappa M, and Cianfarani S. (2016) Water Balance and 'Salt Wasting' in the First Year of Life: The Role of Aldosterone-Signaling Defects. Horm Res Paediatr. 86: 143-153. DOI:10.1159/000449057.

[31] Neville M. (1990). The physiological basis of milk secretion. Ann N Y Acad Sci. 586:1-11. DOI:10.1111/

j.1749-6632.1990.tb17783.x. PMID: 2192630.

[32] Myatt L, and Roberts J. (2015) Preeclampsia: Syndrome or Disease. Curr Hypertens Rep. 17: 83. DOI: 10.1007/s11906-015-0595-4.

[33] Poon L and Nicolaides K. (2014) Early Prediction of Pre-eclampsia. Obstetrics and Gynecology International: article ID 297397. DOI: 10.1155/2014/297397.

[34] Costa F. Murth P, Keogh R, and Woodrow N. (2011) Early Screening for preeclampsia. The Revista Brasileira de Ginecologia e Obstetr'ıci 367–375.

[35] Ogge G, Chaiworapongsa T, Romero R, Hussein Y, Kusanovic J, Yeo L, Kim C, and Hassan S. (2011). Placental Lesions Associated with Maternal Underperfusion are more Frequent in Early-onset than in Late-onset Pre-eclampsia. J Perinat Med 39: 641-652. 25. DOI:10.1515/JPM.2011.098.

[36] Morente J, Cacas-David I, Penolino V. (2018). Association of hypokalemia and preeclampsia and correlation of serum potassium to blood pressure severity in preeclampsia. Philippine Journal of Obstetrics and Gynecology. 42: (2013). 9-16.

[37] Sayyed A, Sonttake A. Electrolyte status in preeclampsia. Online International Interdisciplinary Research Journal. 3(3) 30-33.

[38] Estabrook G, Brown M, & Sargent I. (2011) The origins and end-organ consequence of pre-eclampsia. Best Practice and Research Clinical Obstetrics and Gynaecology. 25: 435-447.

[39] Lupoglazoff J, Jacoz-Aigrain E, Guyot B, Chappey O, and Blot P. (1993) Endogenous digoxin-like immunoreactivity during pregnancy and at birth. Br J clin Pharmac. 35: 251-254.

[40] Redman C, Sargent I, Staff A. (2014). IFPA Senior Award Lecture: Making sense of pre-eclampsia – Two placental causes of preeclampsia. Placenta. DOI:10.1016/j.placenta.2013.12.008.

[41] Reis F, D'Antona, Petraglia F. (2002). Predictive Value of Hormone Measurements in Maternal and Fetal Complications of Pregnancy. (2002). Endocrine Reviews. 23: 230-257.

[42] Grill S, Rusterholz C, Zanetti-Dallenbach R, Tercanli S, Holzgreve W, Hahn S, Lapaire O. (2009) Potential markers of preeclampsia – a review. Reproductive Biology and Endocrinology. 7:70. DOI:10.1186/1477-7827-7-70.

[43] Myatt L, Miodovnik M. (1999). Prediction of Preeclampsia. Seminars in Perinatology 23: 45-57.

[44] Grill S, Rusterholz C, Zanetti-Dallenbach R, Tercanli S, Holzgreve W, Hahn S, Lapaire O. (2009). Potential markers of preeclampsia – a review. Reproductive Biology and Endocrinology. 7:70. DOI:10.1186/1477-7827-7-70

[45] Alberry M, Bills V, Soothill P. (2011). Review: An update on pre-eclampsia prediction research. The Obstetrician and Gynaecologist. 13: 79-85.

[46] Suzuki H, Ohkuchi A, Shirasuna K, Takahashi H, Usui R, Matsubara S, Suzuki M. (2014). Animal Models of Preeclampsia: Insight into Possible Biomarker Candidates for Predicting Preeclampsia. Med J. Obstet Gynecol. 2 (2): 1031.

[47] Sunderland N, Hennessy A, Makris A. (2011). Animal Models of Pre-eclampsia. Am J of Reproductive Immunology 65: 533-541.

[48] Larre A, Parisotto A, Rockenbach B, Pasin D, Capellari C, Escouto C, da

Costa B, Poli-de-Figueredo C. (2017). Phosphodiesterases and preeclampsia. Medical Hypotheses 108:94-100. DOI: 10.1016/j.mehy.2017.08.003

[49] Trapani A, Goncalves L, Trapani T, Viera S, Pires M, deSouza Pires, M. (2016). Perinatal and Hemodynamic Evaluation of Sildenafil Citrate for Preeclampsia Treatment: A Randomized Clinical Trial. Obstet Gynecol 128: 253-259. DOI:10.1097/ AOG.0000000000001518.

[50] Podymow T, August P. (2007). Update on the Use of Antihypertensive Drugs in Pregnancy. Hypertension. 51: 960-969. DOI:10.1161/ HYPERTENSIONAHA.106.075895

[51] Adair C, Luper A, Rose J, Russell G, Veille J, Buckalew V. (2009). The hemodynamic effects of intravenous digoxin-binding fab immunoglobulin in severe pre-eclampsia: a double-blind, randomized, clinical trial. Journal of Perinatology. 29: 284-289.

[52] Puschett J, Aguanne E, Uddin M. (2010). Marinobufagenin, resibufogenin and preclampsia. Biochimica et Biophysica Acta. 1802 1246-1253. DOI:10.1016/j. bbadis.2010.02.005.

[53] Abi-Ghanem D, Lai X, Berghman L, Horvat D, Li J, Ro, o D, Uddin M, Kamano Y, Npgawa T, Xu J, Pettit G, Puschett. (2011). A chemifluorescent immunoassay for the determination of marinobufagenin in body fluids. J Immunoassay Immunochem. 32: 31-46 DOI:10.1080/15321819.2010. 538107

[54] Agunanne E, Horvat D, Harrison R, Uddin M, Jones R, Kuehl T, Ghanem D, Berghman L, Lai X, Li J, Romo D, Puschett J. (2010). Marinobufagenin Levels in Preeclamptic Patients: A Preliminary Report. Am J Perinatology. DOI:10.1055/s-0031-1272965. ISSN 0735-1631.

[55] Fedorva L, Raju V, El-Okdi N, Shidyak A, Kennedy D, Vetteth S, Giovannucci D, Bagrov A, Fedorva O, Shapiro J, Malhotra D. The cardiotonic steroid hormone marinobufagenin induces renal fibrosis: implication of epithelialto-mesenchymal transition. Am J Physiol Renal Physiol (2009) 296: F922-F934. DOI:10.1152/ ajprenal.90605.2008

[56] Fedorova O, Tapilskaya N, Bzhelyansky A, Frolova E, Nikitina E, Reznik V, Kashkin V, Bagrov A. (2010). Interaction of Digibind with endogenous cardiotonic steroids from preclamptic placentae. J Hypertens. 28: 361-366. DOI:10.1097/ HJH.0b01328333226c.

[57] Fedorova O, Simbirtsen A, Kolodkin N, Kotov A, Agalakova N, Kashkin V, Tapliskaya N, Bzhelyansky A, Reznik V, Frolova E, Nokitina E, Budny G, Longo D, Lakatta E, Bagrov A. (2008). Monoclonal antibody to an endogenous bufadienolide, marinobufagenin, reverses preeclampsia-induced Na/K-ATPase inhibition and lowers blood pressure in NaCl-sensitive hypertension. J Hypertens. 26(12): 2414-2425. DOI:10.1097/ HJH.0b013e328312c86a.

Section 2

Factors Affecting Preeclampsia

Chapter 2

Role of Vitamin D in Preeclampsia

Simmi Kharb

Abstract

Pathogenesis of preeclampsia involves immune dysfunction, placental implantation, abnormal angiogenesis, excessive inflammation, hypertension that may be affected by vitamin D. Human placenta expresses all the components for vitamin D signaling: Vitamin D receptor (VDR), retinoid X receptor (RXR), 1-alpha- hydroxylase (CYP27B1) and 24- hydroxylase (CYP24A1). Vitamin D binding protein plays a role in binding and transportation of 25 hydroxyvitamin D [25(OH)D] and 1,25$(OH)_2D_3$. Vitamin D is activated by 25-hydroxylase (CYP2R1) and 1-alpha -hydroxylase (CYP27B1) and is degraded by 24-hydroxylase (CYP24A1). Vitamin D supplementation is not recommended by WHO for pregnant women and allows recommended nutrient intake (RNI) of 200 IU (5 μg) per day. Further research requires serum 25(OH)D analysis and assessment of maternal and infant outcomes; pre-conceptional vitamin D status.

Keywords: Vitamin D, vitamin D receptor, cytochrome P450, pregnancy, preeclampsia, cord blood

1. Introduction

Pathogenesis of preeclampsia involves immune dysfunction, placental implantation, abnormal angiogenesis, excessive inflammation, hypertension that may be affected by vitamin D [1]. Preeclampsia complicates 2–8% of pregnancies globally and the incidence continues to increase worldwide. Preeclampsia (PE) is associated with significant maternal morbidity and mortality.

2. Pathogenesis of preeclampsia

Numerous pathophysiologic abnormalities have been suggested to explain the mechanisms of the origin of preeclampsia. Despite intensive research efforts, the etiology and pathogenesis of PE are not completely understood. The development of preeclampsia is influenced by genetic, immunologic, and environmental risk factors suggesting a multifactorial origin. Currently, there is no single reliable, cost-effective screening test for preeclampsia. A baseline laboratory evaluation is performed early in pregnancy in women who are at high risk for preeclampsia.

It is obvious that no single mechanism is responsible for this syndrome. The initiating abnormality is failed vascular remodeling of the vessels that supply the placental bed (stage 1). This was linked to the maternal syndrome of preeclampsia (stage 2). Two key features in the pathogenesis of preeclampsia are shallow endovascular cytotrophoblast invasion in the spiral arteries and endothelial cell dysfunction.

According to Barker's theory (also, called fetal programming or fetal origins of disease), origin of some adulthood chronic diseases such as cardiovascular diseases, hypertension and diabetes have their origin in intrauterine life. This hypothesis suggests that the intrauterine environment in which the fetus develops may be responsible for complications in adult life. Changes occurring in intrauterine environment and that somehow could disrupt normal development of the fetus can trigger metabolic changes, which may result in the development of long-term disorders. Preeclampsia has implications for future pregnancies and future cardiovascular risk.

3. Vitamin D metabolism during pregnancy

Since fetus completely relies on the maternal stores for its growth and development, vitamin D status during pregnancy has an important effect on this. During early pregnancy, 1,25$(OH)_2$D increases and they continue to increase until delivery. This increase in 1,25$(OH)_2$D is dependent on the available 25(OH)D levels and are independent of calcium metabolism (**Figure 1**).

The primary role of vitamin D in pregnancy is immunomodulatory in addition to its classical calcium regulatory function. According to Barker's hypothesis, the developmental origins of adult disease lie mainly in prenatal factors such as nutritional insults occurring during pregnancy and/or early infancy period [2].

Vitamin D metabolism during pregnancy and fetal development is different as compared with non-pregnant state, The conversion of vitamin D to 25(OH)D is unchanged during pregnancy. The conversion of 25(OH)D to 1,25$(OH)_2$D during pregnancy is unique and unparalleled during life and at no other time during life 25(OH)D is so closely linked with 1,25$(OH)_2$D production.

During pregnancy, the rise in 1,25$(OH)_2$D in the mother and fetus is dependent on substrate availability i.e., 25(OH)D, and this is largely independent of calcium

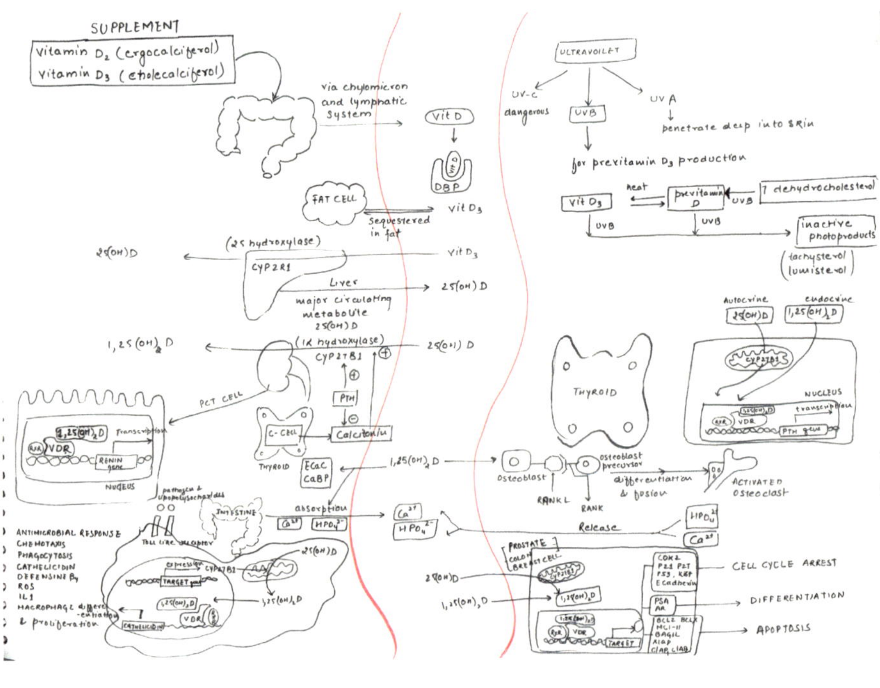

Figure 1.
Overview of vitamin D metabolism, its role and mechanism of action.

homeostasis. The 1,25$(OH)_2$D serum concentrations double by 12th weeks of gestation and continue to rise two- to threefold from the non-pregnant baseline rising (to over 700 pmol·L^{-1}) attaining levels that would be toxic due to hypercalcemia to the non-pregnant individual, but which are essential during pregnancy. Neither in the mother nor in the fetus during the pregnant state, this conversion seems to be controlled by classic calcium homeostatic mechanisms. Calcium homeostasis, however, is not linked with this increase in 1,25$(OH)_2$D, because there is no increase in calcium demand by either the mother or fetus at 12 weeks of gestation. In contrast, the increased 1,25$(OH)_2$D levels remain sustained during pregnancy and during lactation these levels are not sustained when the maternal calcium demands are high.

The mechanism of uncoupling of calcium metabolism from 1,25$(OH)_2$D generation during pregnancy and not lactation is not clear. It could be due to the fact that 1,25$(OH)_2$D is an important immune modulator involved in maternal tolerance to the foreign fetus since pregnant women with preeclampsia have a clinical picture of inflammation and vasculitis, vitamin D deficiency has been implicated and vitamin D is a known modulator of inflammation [3].

Experimental animal studies have also strongly shown that vitamin D deficiency is a potential mechanism of placental dysfunction and respiratory maturation [4].

There is disruption of endothelial stability and an enhancement of "vascular leak" during preeclampsia and experimental animal models of preeclampsia have clearly demonstrated that endothelial instability leads to placental ischemia [5].

Vitamin D_3,25(OH)D_3 and 1,25$(OH)_2D_3$ stabilize endothelium and endothelium "leak" through non-genomic mechanisms and on equal molar basis, vitamin D_3 has more potent action as compared to 25(OH)D_3 or 1,25$(OH)_2$D. Vitamin D_3 is the most accessible form for cell membrane and it exists mainly bound to VDBP in circulation and only miniscule amount of vitamin D_3 exist in the free form. Vitamin D_3 has a longer half-life following its endogenous synthesis (in skin) as compared to the exogenous vitamin D taken orally and the half-life of 25(OH)D is weeks. Vitamin D_3 when given at physiological doses of 4 000 IU·d^{-1} or greater circulates in the "free" form at significant levels to be available to membrane insertion and subsequent endothelial stabilization that is likely to have profound effects on several disease processes. Recent studies have implicated maternal vitamin D deficiency as a risk factor for abnormal fetal growth patterns, adverse birth outcomes, increased risk of preterm birth. and reproductive failure [6, 7].

1,25-dihydroxyvitamin D [1,25$(OH)_2$D] is primary bioactive form, and it does not readily cross the placenta, umbilical cord concentrations of its precursor, 25(OH) D, are similar to maternal concentrations. Placenta modulates circulating vitamin D metabolites in pregnant women and favors the uptake of DBP-bound 25(OH)D_3 through a specific receptor system (LRP2-CUBN) and has CYP27B1 activity.

Both maternal decidua and fetal trophoblast have detectable CYP27B1 activity and they express VDR. Placental production of 1,25$(OH)_2$D has been documented to be essential for immunosuppressive effects required for immune tolerance of implantation. Vitamin D may have a more extensive role in placental function, including trophoblastic differentiation and extravillous trophoblast invasion of the decidua and myometrium and a fundamental role in the process of conception, implantation and development of the placenta itself. However, the precise role of vitamin D in the process of implantation remains unclear.

Studies have shown that 1,25$(OH)_2$D regulates homeobox gene HOXA10 expression in human endometrial stromal cells which is important for the development of endometrial development and implantation. Animal studies have shown that female rats on a vitamin D-deficient diet had overall reduction of fertility and failure of implantation and administration of 1,25$(OH)_2$D corrected this.

In addition, vitamin D via its immunomodulatory actions may also influence implantation indirectly. Decidual synthesis of 1,25$(OH)_2$D has the potential to influence uterine natural killer cells, dendritic cells, macrophages and T-cells throughout pregnancy, including inhibition of Th1 cytokines and promotion of Th2 cytokines, that have a significant role in the process of implantation [8].

Obesity is also a major contributing factor to vitamin D status in pregnant women that causes lowering of 25(OH)D levels in pregnant women with high body mass index (BMI).

4. Vitamin D signaling in pregnancy

Vitamin D signaling is important for normal placental function and fetal growth. Vitamin D maintains healthy cellular functions and redox and Ca^{2+} signaling systems and increases expression of both Nrf2 and the anti-aging protein Klotho, a major regulator of Ca^{2+} and redox signaling. Declining vitamin D levels reduces the stability of this regulatory signaling network and may cause many of the major diseases linked to vitamin D deficiency which are associated with a dysregulation in both ROS and Ca^{2+} signaling [9].

Also, vitamin D signaling depends on availability and turnover of active vitamin D receptor (VDR) ligand 1,25-dihydroxycholecalciferol and efficiency of VDR transactivation. Net availability of active hormone depends on the delivery of substrate and the balance of activating and inactivating enzymes, mainly secosteroid metabolizing p450 enzymes (e.g., various hydroxylase enzymes: 25 hydroxylase, 24 hydroxylase and 1- alpha hydroxylase). Out of these hydroxylases, 1- alpha hydroxylase is expressed in kidney and released in systemic circulation to serve as a critical activating enzyme in circulation. It is also synthesized in target tissues and activates local secosteroid. 1- alpha hydroxylase in kidney is upregulated by low calcium intake and parathyroid hormone inactivates both phosphatonins [10] as well as proinflammatory signal transduction downregulates its expression.

Transactivation of VDR depends on exact molecular structure, nuclear translocation, and presence of heterodimer retinoid X-receptor (RXR) and other nuclear cofactors to regulate gene expression, however, membrane receptor for these effects is not yet identified.

Rickets is a syndrome of impaired vitamin D signaling due to vitamin D_3 deficiency and can be caused by inherited defects of the cascade, nutritional deficits, lack of sunlight exposure, malabsorption, and underlying diseases like chronic inflammation. Vitamin D signaling is complex and modulated at multiple levels.

1,25 $(OH)_2$ D can diffuse freely across the plasma membrane and binds its high-affinity nuclear receptor (VDR, vitamin D receptor) to mediate its effects transcriptionally and post transcriptionally. In the transcriptional pathway, 1,25$(OH)_2$D bind to VDR and forms a heterodimer complex (VDR- RXR complex) with retinoid X receptor (RXR). The VDR-RXR complex binds to vitamin D response element (VDRE) in the promoter region to regulate the target expression of vitamin D. Also, there is non-transcriptional pathway of vitamin D signaling having modulatory effects via binding of calcitriol- VDR complex with caveolae to stimulate signaling cascades namely, protein kinase C and mitogen-activated protein kinase. These signaling cascades regulate various cellular functions such as proliferation, differentiation, invasion, and apoptosis. Altered VDR expressions have been associated with various cancers, however, role of VDR and vitamin D signaling in pregnancy is poorly understood.

5. Vitamin D- induced genomic alterations during pregnancy

Vitamin D supplementation during pregnancy appears to affect genetic information of several highly functional modules related to systemic inflammation and immune responses and implicates the emergence of a distinctive immune response in women destined to develop preeclampsia [11].

Both non-genomic and genomic actions of vitamin D can affect epigenetic regulation of fetal development, and dynamic changes occur in epigenetic markers namely, methylation, hydroxylation, post translational modifications (covalent modifications) various short and long RNAs that regulate the transcriptional gene activity during the acquirement of specific cellular functions. A subset of epigenetics are programmed during early pregnancy that are stably maintained into adulthood [12].

6. Role of vitamin D binding protein (VDBP) in PE

VDBP is plasma carrier protein that binds metabolites of vitamin D to be transported in the body. Vitamin D-binding protein [VDBP, group-specific component (GC) of serum (GC-globulin)] is encoded by the GC gene. VDBP is synthesized mainly in liver and synthesized in adipose tissue, kidneys, and gonads. VDBP is 58 kDa glycosylated alpha-globulin composed of 458 amino acid residues in length and it folds into a triple-domain structure bound by disulphide bonds.

VDBP has immunomodulatory properties and is involved in chemotaxis of fatty acids and endotoxins. Immunological role for VDBP in pre-eclampsia in VDBP of placental origin has been documented as autoimmune target of autoantibodies in the sera of pre-eclamptic women compared with the sera of healthy non-pregnant women. Maternal obesity is associated with adverse health effects for both mother and newborn along with increased inflammation seems to be an important pathological mechanism for detrimental effects of obesity during pregnancy. However, role of vitamin D in the process is still remains to be clarified.

VDBP-macrophage activating factor (DBP-MAF) is involved in bone metabolism. VDBP has been shown to increase drastically during pregnancy as compared to non-pregnant women, reaching their peak in early third trimester and with the lowest level at approximately 36 weeks gestation. This increase is associated with increased total 25(OH)D and decreased free and bioavailable 25(OH)D to increase the capacity to store and metabolize more vitamin D to maintain sufficient concentration of vitamin D throughout pregnancy and lactation to support their increased requirements.

The increase in VDBP during pregnancy could also occur in response to rising estrogen. VDBP has been reported to increase when oestrogens levels are increased in conditions such as high stress states, some ovarian tumors and hormone replacement therapies.

Fetus obtains its supply of vitamin D via placenta which has also been shown to express VDBP. Placental cells express the components of vitamin D signaling including VDR and VDBP and can synthesize and respond to $1,25(OH)_2D_3$ and $24,25(OH)_2D$. The maternal vitamin D compounds may enter the placental cells by endocytosis of 25(OH)D-VDBP and/or by diffusion of the free hormone to be transformed into $1,25(OH)_2D_3$ or $24,25(OH)_2D$, however, the exact mechanism is not known. Without VDBP maternally derived 25(OH)D may not enter placental cells and its transformation into the active form of vitamin D and its transport to the fetus for utilization would not be possible.

SNPs of three genes involved in vitamin D metabolism including GC have been implicated in pre-eclampsia risk. GC-1 phenotype has been identified as a genetic marker for early detection for women at risk of pre-eclampsia. This has been shown that in South African (HIV endemic region) pregnant women complicated by pre-eclampsia that two SNPs of GC gene (rs4588 and rs7041) are more frequently present.

Status of VDBP and total 25(OH)D in preeclampsia is still not clear. Few studies have reported that different VDBP plasma concentrations in women who developed pre-eclampsia as compared to pregnant normotensive controls and no correlations have been noted between VDBP and total 25(OH)D. The increased oxidative stress in pregnancy may be responsible for the altered concentration of VDBP and vitamin D metabolism in placentae in preeclampsia. Moreover, proteinuria in preeclampsia have been shown to cause urinary loss of VDBP as compared to normotensive pregnancies possibly due to disruption of vitamin D metabolism and function through reduced VDBP.

Current evidence suggests that VDBP has been implicated in pregnancy, but its exact role is not yet fully understood. More focused studies are needed to address these limitations to disentangle the functions of VDBP and to clarify its role as a measure of vitamin D status and an important novel biomarker of pregnancy and reproductive outcomes.

7. Role of cytochrome P450 in PE

Two hepatic P450 enzymes catalyzing 25-hydroxylation of vitamin D_3 (VD_3) exist in mammalian liver namely, mitochondrial, and microsomal enzymes. Mitochondrial vitamin D_3 25-hydroxylase is apparently identical with CYP27A.

VD_3 is activated to 1α,25-dihydroxyvitamin D3 (1,25-D_3) by cytochrome P450 2R1 (CYP2R1)/CYP27A1 and CYP27B1 (1-alpha-hydroxylase) sequentially and deactivated by multiple enzymes including CYP3A4. 1,25-D_3 can activate the transcription of CYP3A genes. Activated vitamin D receptor (VDR) forms a heterodimer with retinoid X receptor α (RXRα) to recruit co-activators and translocate this to the nucleus for its binding to specific vitamin D responsive elements (VDRE), and thus activates the gene transcription. This transactivation effect modulates the nutrient bioavailability and drug metabolism. Also, extrarenal expression of CYP27B1 (1-alpha-hydroxylase) generates 1,25$(OH)_2$D in numerous target tissues including the placenta and brain. Vitamin D receptor (VDR) regulates cytochrome P450 3A (CYP3A) expression in human and VDR-response elements are found in the promoter region of CYP3A genes [13].

8. Vitamin D supplementation in pregnancy

Vitamin D dysregulation during pregnancy has been linked to adverse effects on placental function and pregnancy and there is requirement for adequate vitamin D status across gestation. Pregnant women are at high risk of vitamin D deficiency (VDD) and VDD during pregnancy is associated with increased risk of gestational diabetes and preeclampsia. Since preeclampsia can affect offspring health resulting in low birth weight, poor skeletal health, impaired brain development, autoimmune disease, obesity, and insulin resistance.

Randomized controlled trials investigating vitamin D supplementation during pregnancy have revealed that increased vitamin D supplementation decreased complications of pregnancy and C-section births and improve birth outcome data.

Recent randomized controlled trials involving vitamin D supplementation in high-risk pregnancies have demonstrated decreased cesarean section rate and maternal hospitalization, decreased macrosomia and hospitalization in newborns of women with gestational diabetes. Favorable effects on insulin metabolism parameters, serum HDL cholesterol and total cholesterol concentrations in women with pre-eclampsia risk factors were also reported [14].

9. WHO recommendations

Vitamin D supplementation is not recommended for pregnant women to improve maternal and perinatal outcomes [15].

Remarks:

- These recommendation do not propose any alterations in the prevalent WHO recommendation regarding vitamin D supplementation during pregnancy as per WHO ANC guidelines.
- According to WHO guidelines on healthy eating, the pregnant women should receive adequate nutrition and consumption of healthy, balanced diet, according to WHO guidance on healthy eating during pregnancy.
- Since sunlight is one of important source of vitamin D and it is not known that how much duration of sunlight is required. This depends on various variables namely, amount of skin being exposed to sunlight, time of day, altitude and seasonal variations, pigmentation of skin (in darker skin, less vitamin D is synthesized by pigments are synthesized as compared to lighter pigments) and sunscreen use also decreases its production.
- In the cases of documented vitamin D deficiency or in pregnant women, vitamin D supplements may be given as per the guidelines of WHO

*This is an extract from the relevant guideline (https://www.who.int/publications-detail-redirect/9789240008120).

10. Future research

The complexity of vitamin D metabolism and functions involved in placental development are still to be fully elucidated and they are likely to be a key component of future studies of vitamin D in pregnancy. Further studies of vitamin D and adverse events in early pregnancy are required.

This needs to be clarified in future studies that how variations in vitamin D system in placenta and fetal trophoblast cells can affect implantation and regulate maintenance of a successful healthy pregnancy.

Role of vitamin D in maternal obesity is still not clear. Only a limited number of reports of vitamin D deficiency and miscarriage are available, and such studies need to be expanded by including more rigorous supplementation trials.

The mechanism of alteration of offspring epigenetic status by maternal VDD and the physiological impact of these epigenetic modifications remains uncertain. Future studies are needed to elucidate the mechanism and searching the windows for effective timely intervention via supplementation. Since VDD critically affects developmental programming of short- and long-term offspring metabolic and neurobehavioral health, potentially via epigenetic mechanisms, exploration of mechanisms of non-genomic or genomic effects of vitamin D is required.

11. Conclusions

A proper understanding of causal mechanisms that lead to adverse health in offspring born to VDD mothers is required for early diagnoses and improving treatment during pregnancy so as to prevent later adverse DOHaD (developmental origins of adult disease) effects in at-risk offspring and mothers in future. Some genetic variants of VDBP have also been reported to be associated with these adverse outcomes. Further studies are required to explore more accurate VDBP assays and exploring ethnic variation and potential confounders are needed to clarify whether VDBP is associated with reproductive health and pregnancy outcomes, and the mechanisms underlying these relationships and possible role of vitamin D during pregnancy to prevent adverse fetal and maternal outcome.

Acknowledgements

Special thanks to my teachers, students and patients for inspiring me.

Conflict of interest

None. There is no conflict of interest.

Notes/thanks/other declarations

None.

Author details

Simmi Kharb
Department of Biochemistry, MRU, Pt. B.D. Sharma PGIMS, Pt. B.D. Sharma UHS, Rohtak, Haryana, India

*Address all correspondence to: simmikh@gmail.com

References

[1] Bruce W Hollis, Carol L Wagner. New insights into the vitamin D requirements during pregnancy. Bone Res 2017; 5: 17030 doi: 10.1038/boneres.2017.30.

[2] Heaney RP. Is Vitamin D Inadequacy in Early Life an Instance of the "Barker Hypothesis"? Nutr Today 2016 ;51: 14-17.

[3] Bodnar LM, Simhan HN, Catov JM, Roberts JM, Platt RW, Diesel JC, Klebanoff MA. Maternal vitamin D status and the risk of mild and severe preeclampsia. Epidemiology 2014; 25:207-214.

[4] Faulkner JL, Cornelius DC, Amaral LM, Harmon AC, Cunningham MW Jr, Darby MM, Ibrahim T, Thomas DS, Herse F, Wallukat G, Dechend R, LaMarca B. Vitamin D supplementation improves pathophysiology in a rat model of preeclampsia. Am J Physiol Regul Integr Comp Physiol 2016; 310:R346-R354.

[5] LaMarca B, Amaral LM, Harmon AC, Cornelius DC, Faulkner JL, Cunningham MW Jr. Placental ischemia and resultant phenotype in animal models of preeclampsia. Curr Hypertens Rep 2016; 18:38. doi: 10.1007/s11906-016-0650-9.

[6] Pal L, Zhang H, Williams J, Santoro NF, Diamond MP, Schlaff WD, Coutifaris C, et al. Vitamin D status relates to reproductive outcome in women with polycystic ovary syndrome: secondary analysis of a multicenter randomized controlled trial. J Clin Endocrinol Metab 2016; 101:3027-3035.

[7] Kiely ME, Zhang JY, Kinsella M, Khashan AS, Kenny LC. Vitamin D status is associated with uteroplacental dysfunction indicated by pre-eclampsia and small-for-gestational-age birth in a large prospective pregnancy cohort in Ireland with low vitamin D status. Am J Clin Nutr 2016 ;104:354-361.

[8] Ganguly A, Tamblyn JA, Finn-Sell S, Chan SY, Westwood M, Gupta J, et al. Vitamin D, the placenta and early pregnancy: effects on trophoblast function. J Endocrinol 2018 ;236: R93-R103.

[9] Michael J. Berridge. Vitamin D cell signalling in health and disease, Biochem Biophys Res Commun 2015; 460: 53-71.

[10] Ebert R, Schütze N, Adamski J, Jakob F. Vitamin D signaling is modulated on multiple levels in health and disease. Mol Cell Endocrinol 2006; 248:149-159.

[11] Schulz EV, Cruze L, Wei W, Gehris J, Wagner CL. Maternal vitamin D sufficiency and reduced placental gene expression in angiogenic biomarkers related to comorbidities of pregnancy. J Steroid Biochem Mol Bio. 2017; 17:273-279.

[12] Suderman M, Stene LC, Bohlin J, Page CM, Holvik K, Parr CL, , et al. 25-Hydroxyvitamin D in pregnancy and genome wide cord blood DNA methylation in two pregnancy cohorts (MoBa and ALSPAC). J Steroid Biochem Mol Biol 2016;159:102-109.

[13] Xuan Qin, Xin Wang, Sinica B. Role of vitamin D receptor in the regulation of CYP3A gene expression. Acta Pharmaceutica 2019;9: 1087-1098.

[14] Karamali M, Beihaghi E, Mohammadi AA, Asemi Z. Effects of high dose vitamin D supplementation on metabolic status and pregnancy outcomes in pregnant women at risk for pre-eclampsia. Horm Metab Res 2015; 47: 867-872.

[15] Nutritional interventions update: vitamin D supplements during pregnancy. WHO antenatal care recommendations for a positive pregnancy experience. 29 July 2020. https://www.who.int/publications-detail-redirect/9789240008120.

Section 3

Cellular Function

Chapter 3

Cellular Functions of ER Chaperones in Regulating Protein Misfolding and Aggregation: An Emerging Therapeutic Approach for Preeclampsia

Janaranjani Murugesan, Ajithkumar Balakrishnan, Premkumar Kumpati and Hemamalini Vedagiri

Abstract

Proteinuria is one of the hallmarks of preeclampsia (PE) that differentiates other hypertensive disorders of pregnancy. Protein misfolding and aggregation is an emerging pathological condition underlying many chronic metabolic diseases and neurodegenerative diseases. Recent studies indicate protein aggregation as an emerging biomarker of preeclampsia, wherein several proteins are aggregated and dysregulated in the body fluids of preeclamptic women, provoking the multi-systemic clinical manifestations of the disease. At the cellular level, these misfolded and aggregated proteins are potentially toxic interfering with the normal physiological process, eliciting the unfolded protein response (UPR) pathway activators in the endoplasmic reticulum (ER) that subsequently augments the ER quality control systems to remove these aberrant proteins. ER resident chaperones, folding enzymes and other proteins serve as part of the ER quality control machinery in restoring nascent protein folding. These ER chaperones are crucial for ER function aiding in native protein folding, maintaining calcium homeostasis, as sensors of ER stress and also as immune modulators. Consequently, ER chaperones seems to be involved in many cellular processes, yet the association is expanding to be explored. Understanding the role and mechanism of ER chaperones in regulating protein misfolding and aggregation would provide new avenues for therapeutic intervention as well as for the development of new diagnostic approaches.

Keywords: ER stress, ER chaperone, protein misfolding, aggregation, preeclampsia

1. Introduction

Hypertensive disorders are a most common medical problem encountered during pregnancy, affecting 6–8% of all pregnancies. Approximately 70% of hypertensive disorders in pregnancy are mainly due to gestational hypertension, adding up further complications. Preeclampsia (PE) is a multi-systemic disease diagnosed by the presence of new onset hypertension accompanied by proteinuria, renal insufficiency, pulmonary edema, liver failure, neurological complications and fetal growth restriction [1]. The progression of the disease is unpredictable mainly leading to fetal damage associated with other clinical manifestations such as thrombocytopenia, oxidative stress, vascular endothelial dysfunction, systemic inflammation and aberrant angiogenesis, which invariably necessitates early diagnosis of the disease condition so as to prevent further pathogenesis [2].

Proteinuria is one of the hallmarks of preeclampsia that differentiates it from other hypertensive disorders of pregnancy. Recent studies have indicated that protein aggregation as an emerging biomarker of PE, providing insights for therapeutic intervention and development of new diagnostic approaches. Notably, endoplasmic reticulum (ER) stress has recently emerged as a major pathological condition underlying chronic metabolic diseases such as diabetes, cancer, neurodegenerative diseases including PE. At the cellular level, misfolded proteins in the ER significantly lead to ER stress by activating the unfolded protein response (UPR) pathway and molecular chaperones [3–8]. Mis-folded or aggregated proteins are potentially cytotoxic, and consequently cells possess quality control systems to remove these aberrant proteins. These aberrant proteins will expose hydrophobic regions, free cysteines and tend to aggregate, molecular chaperones play key roles in ER quality control because they recognize mis-folded and aggregation-prone proteins [9, 10]. ER chaperones, folding enzymes and other proteins involved in ER stress would serve as a valuable tool in the investigation of disease pathogenesis, prediction of early diagnostic markers and development of targeted therapies. Hence, exploring the structure and functions of ER chaperones would provide new insights in reducing the cellular stress underlying preeclampsia.

2. Regulation of ER stress

Endoplasmic reticulum (ER) is a cellular organelle involved in multiple cellular processes required for cell survival and physiological functions. These processes include intracellular calcium homeostasis, protein secretion and lipid biosynthesis [11–13]. ER constantly monitors the level and conformational status of secreted and membrane-related proteins and rapidly activates multiple signaling pathways in response to changes in the quality and quantity of the proteins it processes, levels of reactive oxygen species and metabolic changes. The ER has a specialized environment, including complexes of chaperones and foldases, as well as high fidelity quality controlling mechanisms to ensure the crucial maintenance of ER homeostasis in cells. ER homeostasis is a unique equilibrium between the cellular demand for protein synthesis and the ER folding capacity to promote protein transportation and maturation.

The ER lumen is a one-of-a-kind biological environment, wherein cells are flooded with calcium inorder to mediate the active transport of proteins by calcium ATPases. In addition, ER is also concentrated in calcium-dependent chaperones such as glucose-regulated protein, 78 kDa (GRP78), GRP94 and calreticulin, which help in stabilizing protein-folding intermediates. The oxidative environment in the ER lumen is crucial for disulphide bond formation mediated by protein disulphide isomerase (PDI). The di-sulfide bond formation helps in the proper folding of many proteins intended for secretion as well as those expressed on the cell surface. Different post-translational modifications, including glycosylation and lipidation of proteins too occur in the ER [14, 15].

Disparity in ER function leads to a state known as ER stress, which activates a series of evolutionarily conserved signaling pathways collectively referred to as the unfolded protein response (UPR). Triggering of UPR pathways results in three effector functions: adaptation, alarm and apoptosis [16]. Initially the UPR pathway intends to recover the homeostasis and normalize the ER function. The adaptive mechanism is primarily involved in the activation of transcriptional pathways responsible for enhancing the protein folding capacity and ER-assisted degradation (ERAD). Both of these pathways reduce the load of misfolded proteins in ER by refolding the proteins or exporting them to cytosol for degradation. Initial to this, translation of mRNA is inhibited to prevent the entry of the new protein into ER until the activation of genes encoding UPR pathways [17].

3. Unfolded protein response pathway

Accumulation of unfolded proteins trigger an evolutionarily conserved signaling pathway designated as UPR [18, 19]. Three major proteins: inositol requiring enzyme 1α/β (IRE1), PKR-like ER kinase (PERK), and activating transcription factor 6α/β (ATF6) are the key UPR signaling activators [20–22]. These activators are capable of retrotrafficking from ER membrane to cytosol by their unique domain organization. They contain 3 domains: an ER luminal domain (LD), a membrane spanning domain and a cytosolic domain. The LD, either directly or indirectly involved in sensing the misfolded proteins [23]. Type 1 transmembrane proteins PERK and IRE1α possess the domain structure that is similar as ER luminal domain structures and a cytosolic Ser/Thr kinase domain, whereas type II transmembrane protein ATF6α contains a cytosolic cyclic AMP response element-binding protein (CREB)-ATF basic leucine zipper domain. UPR pathway activation involves a reduction in protein synthesis, increased protein folding and transport in the ER, an increase in ER-associated protein degradation and autophagy.

After ER is loaded with unfolded proteins, UPR signaling pathways are not simultaneously activated. Primarily ATF6α and IRE1α activation occurs, with subsequent activation of PERK during chronic ER stress [5, 6]. ATF6α and IRE1α are responsible for the activation of transcriptional pathways that increases the cell's capacity for protein folding, transport and degradation. Adaptive response to the protein misfolding is achieved by ATF6α, which is synthesized as an inactive precursor. The N-terminus is located in cytoplasm and serve as an effector portion which possess DNA-binding and transcriptional activation regions. On the accumulation of unfolded protein in ER, ATF6α travels to the Golgi, and the N-terminal effector portion present in cytosol-bZIP transcription factor is fragmented by S1P and S2P [24]. The fragment induces the genes encoding protein chaperones such as binding immunoglobulin protein (BiP), ER protein 57 (ERp57) and glucose-regulated protein 94 (GRP94), proteins involved in ERAD pathway.

X-box binding protein 1 (XBP1), a transcription factor regulating UPR-associated genes is activated by IRE1 [25, 26]. IRE1 acts as an endonuclease and selectively cleaves the 26-nucleotides from the XBP1u mRNA producing XBP1 spliced mRNA (XBP1s). Activated XBP1s enhances the expression of ER chaperone GRP78, increases the phospholipid biosynthesis and also promotes degradation pathways. Regulated IRE1-dependent decay (RIDD) is also mediated by the activation of IRE1α when the ER protein-folding load is intolerable [27–29]. PERK-eIF2α-ATF4 mediated pathway attenuates the non-essential protein synthesis and increases the antioxidant defense system. PERK phosphorylates eIF2α at Ser51 which temporarily stops the initiation of global mRNA translation. In irony, phosphorylated eIF2α upregulates the translation of mRNA's such as ATF4 to increase the protein transport capacity in the ER [30]. Genes encoding ER chaperone protein, folding enzymes and genes encoding ERAD system are activated by p-eIF2α. The collective activation of the genes leads to revive the ER homeostasis

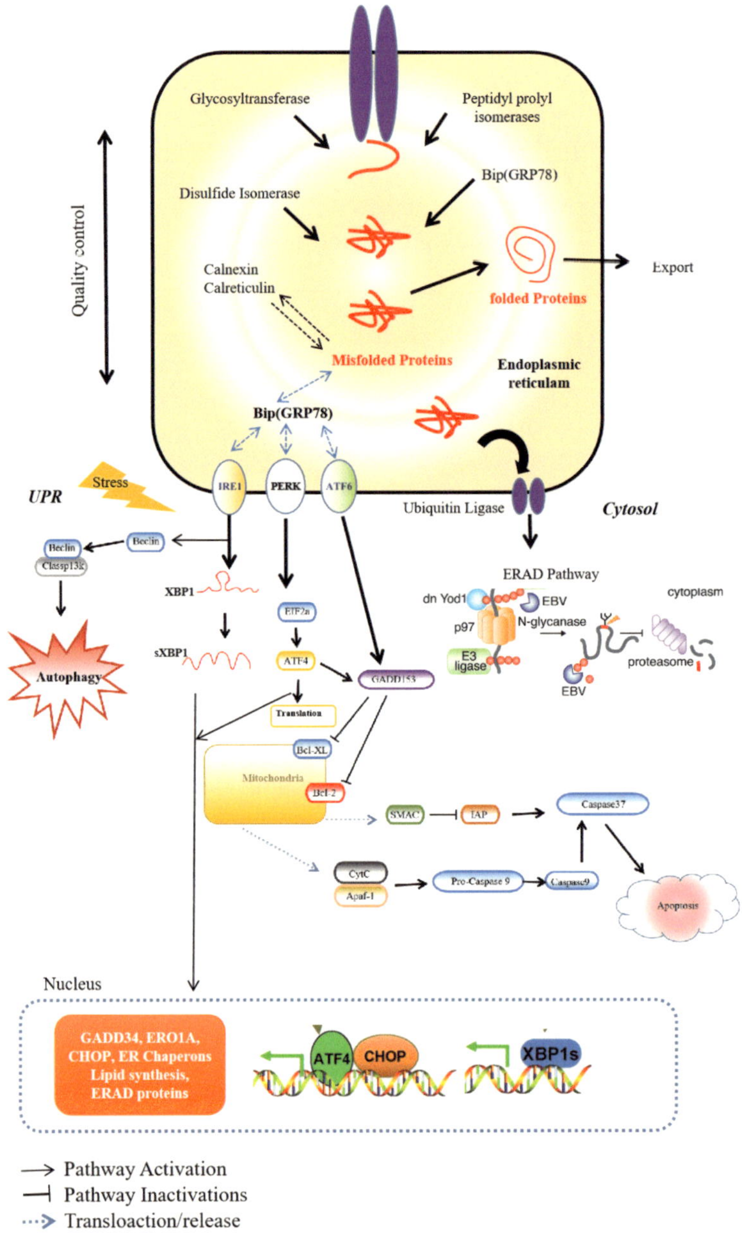

Figure 1.
ER chaperones mediate Protein folding, Quality control, and signaling during ER Stress.

and at saturation, the misfolded proteins are degraded by ERAD system assisted by proteasome mediated degradation and pro-apoptotic protein C/EBP homologous protein (CHOP) [31, 32]. Aforementioned pathways are activated based on the severity of the stress condition (**Figure 1**) [18, 33].

4. Protein misfolding and aggregation

Protein misfolding, aggregation and tissue deposition of fibrous protein aggregates are the critical etiological manifestations of many neurodegenerative diseases such as Alzheimer's disease, Parkinson's disease, Huntington's disease, etc. Recent studies report that numerous aggregated proteins considerably contributes to the heterogeneous clinical manifestations in preeclamptic women, indicating that protein aggregation and misfolding does have a correlation with the disease pathogenesis. Numerous proteomic profiling studies of urine, serum and placental samples from preeclamptic women based on MS analysis, has revealed that aggregation of proteins significantly contributes to the PE associated pathogenesis. Several proteins, including amyloid beta peptide, transthyretin, alpha-1 antitrypsin, albumin, IgG k-free light chains, and ceruloplasmin are aggregated in PE, resulting in toxic deposition of amyloid-like aggregates in the placenta and body fluids [34, 35]. In addition, many extracellular chaperones like casein, clusterin, pregnancy zone protein are implicated to be dysregulated in pregnancy, leading to the accumulation of misfolded proteins and disease manifestation. Probably, these aggregated proteins in the early stages of pregnancy induces defective trophoblast invasion, placental ischemia, ER stress thereby promoting PE manifestation. Insights into the molecular mechanisms of formation of these aggregated proteins and understanding the role of molecular chaperones in regulating the misfolded proteins will open new avenues for pharmacological intervention and therapeutic targeting of PE.

Disruption of ER homeostasis as a result of excess accumulation of unfolded/misfolded proteins due to prolonged or severe ER stress is involved in several pathologies that induce endometriosis and endometrial/ovarian cancers as well as various pregnancy complications that result in preeclampsia, fetal growth restriction and preterm birth. Depending on the severity of ER stress, UPR behaves as sort of binary switch between life and death. Initially, the UPR aims to restore ER homeostasis, but if these attempts fail then the apoptotic cascade is activated. These pathways are now recognized as playing a central role in the pathophysiology of chronic diseases, which contributes to the placental pathology in early-onset PE [36].

The ER has tremendous intracellular store of Ca^{2+} necessary for regulating a variety of cellular functions both in the ER lumen and cytosol. Inside the ER lumen, huge reserves of Ca^{2+} are important for proper protein folding assisting disulfide bond forming chaperone, protein disulfide isomerases (PDI). To maintain the ER calcium levels, sarcoendoplasmic reticulum calcium transport ATPase (SERCA) pumps in the ER membrane actively transport Ca^{2+} from the cytosol into the ER lumen. These pumps are specifically regulated based on the proportion of Ca^{2+} in the ER lumen to the cytosol. Alteration in SERCA pumps blocks the movement of Ca^{2+} into the ER, decreasing the function of molecular chaperones and PDI, thereby increasing the burden of misfolded proteins in the ER [37].

5. Pathophysiology of PE

Impaired placentation mainly contributes to the manifestation of systemic symptoms in PE, which may be preceded or followed by protein misfolding and aggregation along with subsequent placental release of inflammatory cytokines, anti-angiogenetic factors, placental debris and particles as well as protein aggregates into the maternal circulation. This pre-clinical dysregulation causes endothelial dysfunction, excessive thrombin generation, systemic inflammation and as a result, elicits multiorgan syndromes of PE [38–41]. During early stages of pregnancy, several proteins such as transthyretin, may be transported to the placenta from maternal circulation. These aggregation-prone proteins easily undergo misfolding and aggregation in the microenvironment of non-compatible conditions, such as acidic pH, ischemia/hypoxia, amino acid fluctuation, inflammation, and hormonal dysregulation [10, 42]. Protein aggregates induce ER stress and may eventually overwhelm the capacity of the unfolded protein response (UPR) and clearance machineries, leading to deposition and accumulation of these aggregates in trophoblasts, extracellular domains and subsequently causing placental toxicity, poor trophoblast invasion, differentiation, superficial endometrial invasion and failure of spiral artery remodeling. Continuous accumulation of protein aggregates may aggravate ER stress and cause cell apoptosis, leading to release of aggregates into maternal circulation and excretion through injured glomerulus into urine.

ER stress is intricately linked to oxidative stress and inflammation, indicating the co-existence of these pathways in major pathologies particularly early on-set PE, through feed-forward mechanisms [43]. ER stress induction and UPR activation was insignificantly evident in both intra uterine growth retardation (IUGR) and IUGR associated early-onset pre-eclampsia (IUGR + PE) placentas. However, increased apoptosis, higher levels of eIF2α phosphorylation, GRP94 and CHOP in the syncytiotrophoblast and endothelial cells of the foetal capillaries was evident in IUGR + PE placental samples and not in IUGR alone [44]. ER stress associated proteins such as GRP78, GRP94, p-PERK, eIF2α, p-eIF2α, XBP1, CHOP, IRE1, p-IRE1 and inducible nitric oxide synthase (NOS) expression where high in preeclamptic placentas compared to control placenta [45]. Overexpression of placental UPR pathways including IRE1, ATF6 and XBP-1 was significantly observed in early-onset PE compared to that of late-onset of PE and normotensive controls [33]. Preeclamptic placentas feature higher levels of ER stress with prominent activation of pro-inflammatory pathways that contributes to maternal endothelial cell activation. These complexity of cellular responses to ER stress emphasizes the need for a holistic approach for designing potential therapeutic interventions for PE. Antioxidants, ER chaperones, NO donors, statins and H2S donors display pleitropic antioxidant, anti-inflammatory, and pro-angiogenic effects on the signaling pathways involved in the pathophysiology of PE, exhibiting potential strategies for therapeutic intervention [46].

6. ER chaperones

The transcriptional up-regulation of ER chaperones is the hallmark of the ER stress response and occurs in all eukaryotic organisms. The primary function of ER resident chaperones and their cofactors involved in the ER quality control system is to monitor the error-prone steps in protein synthesis and assembly [13, 47]. Three major chaperone families exist in the ER that interact with a wide variety of clients: the lectin chaperones, which generally recognize incompletely folded glycosylated proteins, the heat shock proteins (HSPs) family, which interacts with both nonglycosylated as well as glycosylated proteins and the thiol oxireductases, that aids in the disulphide bond formation [48].

6.1 Heat shock proteins (HSPs)

HSPs are a large family of evolutionarily conserved molecular chaperones, first observed as a group of proteins upregulated in heat-stressed *Drosophila melanogaster* [49], that are well-known for their roles in protein maturation, re-folding and degradation. These molecular chaperones of this HSP family are critical effectors of the UPR adaptive response. They protect intracellular proteins from misfolding or aggregation, inhibit cell death signaling range and preserve the intracellular signaling pathways that are essential for cell survival. HSPs classified according to their molecular weight as proteins of approximately 84 and 70 kDa (HSP84 and HSP70), are amongst the most prominent chaperones in the ER [50]. HSPs are constitutively expressed, inducibly regulated to prevent aggregation of misfolded polypeptides and assists in refolding, besides being crucial modulators of neurotoxicity in Alzheimer's disease [51]. Placental ischemia, oxidative stress, maternal systemic inflammatory response are major elements in the pathogenesis of PE that induces the expression of HSP70 which in-turn is associated with cytokine aggravation, oxidative stress and hepatocellular injury [52].

Binding immunoglobulin protein (BiP)/glucose-regulated protein 78 (GRP78), belongs to the HSP70 family, is a well known ER chaperone that binds to the hydrophobic region of unfolded proteins. GRP78 binds through substrate-binding domain and assists protein folding through a conformational change, achieved through the hydrolysis of ATP by the ATPase domain. Another chaperone, oxygen-regulated protein (ORP)150/GRP170 belonging to the HSP110 family (a HSP70 subfamily), assists the protein folding similar to that of BiP. The group of ER DnaJ proteins-ERdj1, ERdj3/HEDJ, ERdj4, ERdj5, SEC63 and p58IPK belonging to the HSP40 family acts as co-chaperones, mediating the acitivity of BiP by regulating its ATPase activity [53, 54].

Hsp90 is an essential component of cytoplasmic Hsp90-Hsp70 chaperone network, responsible for protein folding. Protein emerging from ribosome is initially folded in nascent polypeptide by Hsp70 and then passed to the Hsp90 for later folding. GRP94, the hsp90 family chaperone, hydrolysis the ATP, facilitates protein folding and liable for the maturation of certain oligomeric proteins including Toll-like receptors (**Table 1**) [58].

Chaperone family	ER chaperone	Function
Heat shock proteins		
	GRP78/BiP	Facilitates folding and assembly of proteins, translocates the newly synthesized polypeptides, targets misfolded proteins for ERAD, regulates calcium homeostasis [27].
	GRP94/endoplasmin	Directs the oxidative folding and assembly of several secreted and membrane proteins that mainly contain disulphide bonds.
Lectin chaperones		
	Calnexin	Transmembrane protein binds to glycan residues of nascent polypeptides found in membrane proximal domains and retains substrate proteins in the ER until they are fully mature and their intermediate oligosaccharide is cleaved by glucosidase II [55].
	Calreticulin	Soluble luminal homolog associates with glycans within the ER lumen and interacts with monoglucosylated glycans, trimmed intermediates of N-linked core glycans on nascent glycoproteins [56].
Thiol oxireductases		
	ERp57/PDIA3	Participates in the folding of numerous cysteine-rich glycoproteins as an element of the CNX/CRT cycle [55].
	PDI/PDIA1/P4HB	Assists in redox protein folding via oxidation, multiple thiol-disulphide exchanges, isomerization, reduction activities and is highly specific in its interaction with different substrates [57].
	ERdj5	Catalyzes the removal of non-native disulfides by binding with BiP and ensures the correct folding of proteins entering the secretory pathway or dislocates misfolded proteins to the cytosol for degradation [54].

Table 1.
Classification of ER chaperones and their functional roles.

6.2 Lectin chaperones

A unique aspect of the ER involves glycosylation-assisted folding which is largely mediated by ER resident lectins. There are two calcium-activating chaperones in the ER - calnexin (CNX) and calreticulin (CRT), that associates with glycoproteins and completes the protein folding process [55, 59]. The CNX/CRT cycle is critical part of the ER quality control machinery in monitoring the glycosylation and sugar chain structures in protein folding and assembly. When one glucose residue is attached to the client protein, ER lectins bind to initiate the folding process and later release the protein to UDP-glucose-glycoprotein glucosyltransferase. The disulfide bond isomerase ER protein 57 (ERp57) majorly involved in the CNX/CRT cycle, catalyzes the oxidation and isomerization of the disulfide bonds in glycoproteins. Further, CRT elicits an immune response through the assembly of major histocompatibility complex (MHC) class I molecules for eventual antigen presentation on the cell surface, intended for apoptosis [60].

6.3 Thiol oxireductases

Formation of transient disulfide bonds in the protein folding process are mediated by thiol oxidoreductases and are essential for the activation of the PERK pathway [56]. These are the major proteins that redox control by utilizing catalytic cysteine residues for oxidation or reduction of their substrates. Protein disulphide isomerase (PDI), ERp72, ERp61, GRP58/ERp57, ERp44 and ERp29 are enzymes that mediate the formation of disulphide bonds through oxidizing cysteine residues of nascent proteins. However, most of the thioloxidoreductases act as oxidants [61] and in certain cancer models, ERp57 as well as PERK gets activated in a PDI dependent manner, reducing cancer cell proliferation and sensitizes cancer cells to ionizing radiation [62].

Hsp47 (Serpin H1) is an ER-resident collagen-specific molecular chaperone that is essential for molecular maturation of collagen. Hsp47 binds Yaa-Gly-Xaa-Arg-Gly in triple-helical procollagen in the ER via hydrophobic and hydrophilic interactions. The binding of Hsp47 stabilizes procollagen by preventing unfolding of the triple helix and aggregate formation. Thus, Hsp47 is indispensable for efficient secretion, processing, fibril formation, and deposition of collagen in the extracellular matrix [63]. The chaperone function of Hsp47 is also involved in the deterioration of fibrosis, suggesting Hsp47 as a therapeutic target for fibrotic diseases, including liver, lung and spleen fibrosis. Lipase maturation factor 1 (LMF1) is an ER chaperone that affects ER lipid metabolism through the activation of lipoprotein, hepatic and endothelial lipases [64]. Mutations in LMF1 are associated with severe hypertriglyceridemia caused by deficiency of these lipases.

7. Conclusion

Preeclampsia is the most frequently encountered medical complication in pregnancy that affects 3–7% of pregnant women worldwide, characterized by de novo on-set of hypertension, proteinuria after 20 weeks of gestation, entailing the heterogeneous etiological disease manifestations. Placental dysfunction due to reduced perfusion, trophoblast remodeling, oxidative stress, ER stress and exaggerated inflammatory response are the major factors that contributes to early on-set preeclampsia. Numerous reports substantiate that ER stress, protein misfolding and aggregation are the major inducers behind the etiological manifestations of PE, leading to disease pathogenesis [65, 66]. Furthermore, amyloid fibrous protein aggregates are an emerging biomarker of PE representing amyloid aggregation of amyloid β, transthyretin, immunoglobulin light chains and alpha-1 antitrypsin. These aggregated proteins mediate defective trophoblast invasion and abnormal remodeling of spiral arteries leading to the onset of PE. This unveils new strategies to identify novel biomarkers as well as targets for therapeutic intervention, to alleviate the underlying pathological conditions and decrease the risk of preeclampsia.

Conflict of interest

The authors declare no conflict of interest.

Author details

Janaranjani Murugesan[1], Ajithkumar Balakrishnan[1], Premkumar Kumpati[2] and Hemamalini Vedagiri[1]*

1 Department of Bioinformatics, Bharathiar University, Coimbatore, Tamil Nadu, India

2 Department of Biomedical Science, Bharathidasan University, Tamil Nadu, India

*Address all correspondence to: hemamalini@buc.edu.in

References

[1] Rana S, Lemoine E, Granger JP, Karumanchi SA. Preeclampsia: Pathophysiology, challenges, and perspectives. Circulation Research. 2019;**124**(7):1094-1112. DOI: 10.1161/CIRCRESAHA.118.313276

[2] Shamshirsaz AA, Paidas M, Krikun G. Preeclampsia, hypoxia, thrombosis, and inflammation. Journal of Pregnancy. 2012;**2012**:1-6

[3] Burton GJ, Yung HW, Murray AJ. Mitochondrial-endoplasmic reticulum interactions in the trophoblast: Stress and senescence. Placenta. 2017;**52**: 146-155

[4] Engin F, Hotamisligil GS. Restoring endoplasmic reticulum function by chemical chaperones: An emerging therapeutic approach for metabolic diseases. Diabetes, Obesity & Metabolism. 2010;**2**:108-115

[5] Ozcan L, Tabas I. Role of endoplasmic reticulum stress in metabolic disease and other disorders. Annual Review of Medicine. 2012;**63**:317-328

[6] Oakes SA, Papa FR. The role of endoplasmic reticulum stress in human pathology. Annual Review of Pathology. 2015;**10**:173-194

[7] Garcia-Huerta P, Bargsted L, Rivas A, Matus S, Vidal RL. ER chaperones in neurodegenerative disease: Folding and beyond. Brain Research. 2016;**1648**(Pt B): 580-587

[8] Steegers EA, von Dadelszen P, Duvekot JJ, Pijnenborg R. Pre-eclampsia. Lancet. 2010;**376**(9741):631-644

[9] Redman CW. Preeclampsia: A multi-stress disorder. La Revue de Médecine Interne. 2011;**32**(Suppl. 1): S41-S44

[10] Gerasimova EM, Fedotov SA, Kachkin DV, Vashukova ES, Glotov AS, Chernoff YO, et al. Protein misfolding during pregnancy: New approaches to preeclampsia diagnostics. International Journal of Molecular Sciences. 2019;**20**(24):6183. DOI: 10.3390/ijms20246183

[11] Anelli T, Sitia R. Protein quality control in the early secretory pathway. The EMBO Journal. 2008;**27**:315-327

[12] Pizzo P, Pozzan T. Mitochondria-endoplasmic reticulum choreography: Structure and signaling dynamics. Trends in Cell Biology. 2007;**17**:511-517

[13] Ma Y, Hendershot LM. ER chaperone functions during normal and stress conditions. Journal of Chemical Neuroanatomy. 2004;**28**(1-2):51-65. DOI: 10.1016/j.jchemneu.2003.08.007

[14] Rizzuto R, Duchen MR, Pozzan T. Flirting in little space: The ER/mitochondria Ca^{2+} liaison. Science's STKE. 2004;**2004**:re1

[15] Schroder M, Kaufman RJ. ER stress and the unfolded protein response. Mutation Research. 2005;**569**:29-63

[16] Xu C, Bailly-Maitre B, Reed JC. Endoplamic reticulum stress: Cell life and death decisions. The Journal of Clinical Investigation. 2005;**115**: 2656-2664

[17] Wu J, Kaufman RJ. From acute ER stress to physiological roles of the unfolded protein response. Cell Death and Differentiation. 2006;**13**:374-384

[18] Ron D, Walter P. Signal integration in the endoplasmic reticulum unfolded protein response. Nature Reviews Molecular Cell Biology. 2007;**8**:519-529

[19] Malhotra JD, Kaufman RJ. The endoplasmic reticulum and the unfolded protein response. Seminars in

Cell & Developmental Biology. 2007;**18**:716-731

[20] Cox JS, Shamu CE, Walter P. Transcriptional induction of genes encoding endoplasmic reticulum resident proteins requires a transmembrane protein kinase. Cell. 1993;**73**(6):1197-1206. DOI: 10.1016/0092-8674(93)90648-a

[21] Harding HP, Zhang Y, Ron D. Protein translation and folding are coupled by an endoplasmic-reticulum-resident kinase. Nature. 1999;**397**(6716):271-274. DOI: 10.1038/16729

[22] Haze K, Yoshida H, Yanagi H, Yura T, Mori K. Mammalian transcription factor ATF6 is synthesized as a transmembrane protein and activated by proteolysis in response to endoplasmic reticulum stress. Molecular Biology of the Cell. 1999;**10**(11):3787-3799. DOI: 10.1091/mbc.10.11.3787

[23] Walter P, Ron D. The unfolded protein response: From stress pathway to homeostatic regulation. Science. 2011;**334**(6059):1081-1086. DOI: 10.1126/science.1209038

[24] Shen J, Chen X, Hendershot L, Prywes R. ER stress regulation of ATF6 localization by dissociation of BiP/GRP78 binding and unmasking of Golgi localization signals. Developmental Cell. 2002;**3**(1):99-111. DOI: 10.1016/s1534-5807(02)00203-4

[25] Lee AH, Iwakoshi NN, Glimcher LH. XBP-1 regulates a subset of endoplasmic reticulum resident chaperone genes in the unfolded protein response. Molecular and Cellular Biology. 2003;**23**:7448-7459

[26] Yoshida H, Matsui T, Yamamoto A, Okada T, Mori K. XBP1 mrna is induced by ATF6 and spliced by IRE1 in response to ER stress to produce a highly active transcription factor. Cell. 2001;**107**:881-891

[27] Lee AS. The ER chaperone and signaling regulator GRP78/BiP as a monitor of endoplasmic reticulum stress. Methods. 2005;**35**:373-381

[28] Kim I, Xu W, Reed JC. Cell death and endoplasmic reticulum stress: Disease relevance and therapeutic opportunities. Nature Reviews. Drug Discovery. 2008;**7**:1013-1030

[29] Rutkowski DT, Kaufman RJ. That which does not kill me makes me stronger: Adapting to chronic ER stress. Trends in Biochemical Sciences. 2007;**32**:469-476

[30] Kadowaki H, Nishitoh H. Signaling pathways from the endoplasmic reticulum and their roles in disease. Genes. 2013;**4**:306-333

[31] Michalak M, Gye MC. Endoplasmic reticulum stress in periimplantation embryos. Clinical and Experimental Reproductive Medicine. 2015;**42**:1-7

[32] Bifulco G, Miele C, di Jeso B, Beguinot F, Nappi C, di Carlo C, et al. Endoplasmic reticulum stress is activated in endometrial adenocarcinoma. Gynecologic Oncology. 2012;**125**:220-225

[33] Yung HW, Atkinson D, Campion-Smith T, Olovsson M, Charnock-Jones DS, Burton GJ. Differential activation of placental unfolded protein response pathways implies heterogeneity in causation of early- and late-onset pre-eclampsia. The Journal of Pathology. 2014;**234**: 262-276

[34] Buhimschi IA, Nayeri UA, Zhao G, Shook LL, Pensalfini A, Funai EF, et al. Protein misfolding, congophilia, oligomerization, and defective amyloid processing in preeclampsia. Science Translational Medicine. 2014;**6**:245ra92

[35] Kalkunte SS, Neubeck S, Norris WE, Cheng S-B, Kostadinov S, Vu Hoang D, et al. Transthyretin is dysregulated in

preeclampsia, and its native form prevents the onset of disease in a preclinical mouse model. The American Journal of Pathology. 2013;**183**:1425-1436

[36] Yoshida H. ER stress and diseases. The FEBS Journal. 2007;**274**(3):630-658. DOI: 10.1111/j.1742-4658.2007.05639.x

[37] Mekahli D, Bultynck G, Parys JB, De Smedt H, Missiaen L. Endoplasmic-reticulum calcium depletion and disease. Cold Spring Harbor Perspectives in Biology. 2011;**3**(6):a004317. DOI: 10.1101/cshperspect.a004317

[38] Chaiworapongsa T, Chaemsaithong P, Yeo L, Romero R. Preeclampsia part 1: Current understanding of its pathophysiology. Nature Reviews. Nephrology. 2014;**10**:466-480

[39] Goel A, Rana S. Angiogenic factors in preeclampsia: Potential for diagnosis and treatment. Current Opinion in Nephrology and Hypertension. 2013;**22**:643-650

[40] Redman CW, Sargent IL. Latest advances in understanding preeclampsia. Science. 2005;**308**:1592-1594

[41] Steegers EA, von Dadelszen P, Duvekot JJ, Pijnenborg R. Preeclampsia. Lancet. 2010;**376**:631-644

[42] Cheng SB, Nakashima A, Sharma S. Understanding pre-eclampsia using Alzheimer's etiology: An intriguing viewpoint. American Journal of Reproductive Immunology. 2016;**75**(3):372-381. DOI: 10.1111/aji.12446. Epub 2015 Nov 20

[43] Burton GJ, Yung HW. Endoplasmic reticulum stress in the pathogenesis of early-onset pre-eclampsia. Pregnancy Hypertension. 2011;**1**(1-2):72-78. DOI: 10.1016/j.preghy.2010.12.002

[44] Yung HW, Calabrese S, Hynx D, Hemmings BA, Cetin I, Charnock-Jones DS. Evidence of placental translation inhibition and endoplasmic reticulum stress in the etiology of human intrauterine growth restriction. The American Journal of Pathology. 2008;**173**:451-462

[45] Du L, He F, Kuang L, Tang W, Li Y, Chen D. eNOS/iNOS and endoplasmic reticulum stress-induced apoptosis in the placentas of patients with preeclampsia. Journal of Human Hypertension. 2017;**31**:49-55

[46] Cindrova-Davies T. The therapeutic potential of antioxidants, ER chaperones, NO and H_2S donors, and statins for treatment of preeclampsia. Frontiers in Pharmacology. 2014;**5**:119. DOI: 10.3389/fphar.2014.00119

[47] Halperin L, Jung J, Michalak M. The many functions of the endoplasmic reticulum chaperones and folding enzymes. IUBMB Life. 2014;**66**:318-326. DOI: 10.1002/iub.1272

[48] Guzel E, Arlier S, Guzeloglu-Kayisli O, Tabak MS, Ekiz T, Semerci N, et al. Endoplasmic reticulum stress and homeostasis in reproductive physiology and pathology. International Journal of Molecular Sciences. 2017;**18**(4):792. DOI: 10.3390/ijms18040792

[49] Ikwegbue, Chukwudi P, Revaprasadu N, Kappo AP. Therapeutic potential of heat shock proteins in human inflammation/autoimmune skin diseases: Future directions. In: Asea AAA, Kaur P, editors. Heat Shock Proteins in Inflammatory Diseases. Vol. 22. Cham: Springer; 2020. pp. 1-16. DOI: 10.1007/7515_2020_36

[50] Burdon RH. Heat shock and the heat shock proteins. Biochemical Journal. 1986;**240**(2):313

[51] Meriin AB, Sherman MY. Role of molecular chaperones in neurodegenerative disorders. International Journal of Hyperthermia. 2005;**21**(5):403-419

[52] Saghafi N, Pourali L, Ghanbarabadi VG, Mirzamarjani F, Mirteimouri M. Serum heat shock protein 70 in preeclampsia and normal pregnancy: A systematic review and meta analysis. International Journal of Reproductive BioMedicine. 2018;**16**(1):1

[53] Garrido C, Gurbuxani S, Ravagnan L, Kroemer G. Heat shock proteins: Endogenous modulators of apoptotic cell death. Biochemical and Biophysical Research Communications. 2001;**286**:433-442

[54] Parcellier A, Gurbuxani S, Schmitt E, Solary E, Garrido C. Heat shock proteins, cellular chaperones that modulate mitochondrial cell death pathways. Biochemical and Biophysical Research Communications. 2003;**304**:505-512

[55] Wu Y, Huang X, Zheng Z, Yang X, Ba Y, Lian J. Role and mechanism of chaperones calreticulin and ERP57 in restoring trafficking to mutant HERG A561V protein. International Journal of Molecular Medicine. 2021;**48**(2):1-12

[56] Venkatesan A, Satin LS, Raghavan M. Roles of calreticulin in protein folding, immunity, calcium signaling and cell transformation. In: Cellular Biology of the Endoplasmic Reticulum. Cham: Springer; 2021. pp. 145-162

[57] Parakh S, Atkin JD. Novel roles for protein disulphide isomerase in disease states: A double edged sword? Frontiers in Cell and Developmental Biology. 2015;**3**:30. DOI: 10.3389/fcell.2015.00030

[58] Lackie RE, Maciejewski A, Ostapchenko VG, Marques-Lopes J, Choy WY, Duennwald ML, et al. The Hsp70/Hsp90 chaperone machinery in neurodegenerative diseases. Frontiers in Neuroscience. 2017;**11**:254. DOI: 10.3389/fnins.2017.00254

[59] Moezzi SMI, Mozafari N, Fazel-Hoseini SM, Nadimi-Parashkoohi S, Abbasi H, Ashrafi H, et al. Apolipoprotein J in Alzheimer's disease: Shedding light on its role with cell signaling pathway perspective and possible therapeutic approaches. ACS Chemical Neuroscience. 2020;**11**(24):4060-4072

[60] Graner MW, Lillehei KO, Katsanis E. Endoplasmic reticulum chaperones and their roles in the immunogenicity of cancer vaccines. Frontiers in Oncology. 2015;**4**:379. DOI: 10.3389/fonc.2014.00379

[61] Bocian-Ostrzycka KM, Grzeszczuk MJ, Banaś AM, Jagusztyn-Krynicka EK. Bacterial thioloxidoreductases—From basic research to new antibacterial strategies. Applied Microbiology and Biotechnology. 2017;**101**(10):3977-3989

[62] Kranz P, Sänger C, Wolf A, Baumann J, Metzen E, Baumann M, et al. Tumor cells rely on the thiol-oxidoreductase PDI for PERK signaling in order to survive ER stress. Scientific Reports. 2020;**10**(1):1-11

[63] Ito S, Nagata K. Biology of Hsp47 (Serpin H1), a collagen-specific molecular chaperone. Seminars in Cell & Developmental Biology. 2016;**62**:142-151. DOI: 10.1016/j.semcdb.2016.11.005

[64] Péterfy M. Lipase maturation factor 1: A lipase chaperone involved in lipid metabolism. Biochimica et Biophysica Acta. 2012;**1821**(5):790-794. DOI: 10.1016/j.bbalip.2011.10.006

[65] Wang M, Kaufman RJ. Protein misfolding in the endoplasmic reticulum as a conduit to human disease. Nature. 2016;**529**:326-335. DOI: 10.1038/nature17041

[66] Hetz C, Papa FR. The unfolded protein response and cell fate control. Molecular Cell. 2017;**69**:169-181. DOI: 10.1016/j.molcel.2017.06.017

Section 4

Organ Dysfunction

Chapter 4

Preeclampsia: From Etiopathology to Organ Dysfunction

Nissar Shaikh, Seema Nahid, Firdous Ummunnisa, Ifrah Fatima, Mohamad Hilani, Asma Gul, A. Al Basha, W. Yahia, F. Al Hail, H. Elfil, E. Abdalla, M.M. Nainthramveetil, M.A Imraan, Muhammad Zubair, Sibghatulla Khan, N. Korichi, S. Alkhawaga, H. Ismail, S. Yaqoob and Mashael Abdulrahman M.S. Al Khelaifi

Abstract

Preeclampsia is a hypertensive disorder of pregnancy affecting 6–12% of the population. There are various risk factors for the development of preeclampsia, ranging from advanced maternal age to genetics. The proposed etiologies for preeclampsia are abnormal placentation, immunological intolerance, endothelial damage, and genetic inheritance. The pathogenesis includes endothelial activation and dysfunction leading to vasospasm. Preeclampsia is divided into two stages: asymptomatic and symptomatic stages. Preeclampsia causes multiple organ involvement, namely central nervous system, respiratory, cardiovascular, hematological dysfunction, HELLP (hemolysis elevated liver enzymes, low platelets) syndrome, endocrine, renal, hepatic, and uteroplacental dysfunction. These organ dysfunctions increase morbidity and mortality in preeclamptic pregnant patients.

Keywords: abnormal placentation, etiology, endothelial dysfunction, epidemiology, hypertensive disorders of pregnancy, HELLP syndrome, long-term impact, multiple organ dysfunction, preeclampsia, risk factors, uteroplacental malfunction

1. Introduction

Hypertension is a common pregnancy-specific medical disorder, which is a significant cause of maternal and perinatal mortality [1]. There is disproportionate risk to the mother and fetus for further complications and long-term sequelae.

Preeclampsia is a hypertensive disorder of pregnancy causing multi-organ dysfunction syndrome with placental dysfunction occurring in the latter half of pregnancy, with major cause of maternal morbidity, maternal intensive care admissions, Cesarean section, end-organ damage, and fetal complications.

2. Definition

Preeclampsia is defined as new onset of hypertension with or without proteinuria or new onset hypertension with evidence of end organ dysfunction after 20 weeks gestation or postpartum in a previously normotensive woman [2].

Classification of hypertension in pregnancy by ACOG (American College of Obstetrician and Gynecologist) 2013 task force:

- Preeclampsia
  - Preeclampsia without severe features
  - Severe preeclampsia with severe features

Progress of preeclampsia is divided into two stages:

2.1 Asymptomatic first stage

It occurs early in pregnancy with impaired remodeling of the spiral arteries and abnormal placentation. This failure of normal angiogenesis results in superficial placentation.

2.2 Symptomatic second stage

It presents in late second or third trimester and is characterized by signs and symptoms distinguished by the release of excess of antiangiogenic factor from intervillous space into the maternal circulation, which causes widespread maternal endothelial dysfunction and accentuated systemic inflammatory response specific to each organ system.

3. Epidemiology

It affects 6–12% of all pregnant women worldwide, with preeclampsia in 5–8% of pregnancy [3, 4]. The WHO (World Health Organization) has identified hypertension as the second most common cause of maternal death among the triad of hemorrhage and sepsis [5]. It is responsible for 70,000 maternal deaths (major cause of maternal morbidity and mortality) and 500,000 fetal deaths worldwide every year [5]. Nulliparous women are prone to develop preeclampsia, while older women are at higher risk of chronic hypertension with superimposed preeclampsia.

Hypertension is well known in pregnancy worldwide, including chronic, gestational, and possible dangerous preeclampsia [6]. It is considered as high-risk pregnancy when unfavorable conditions prevail for the well-being of mother, fetus, or both.

Effective antenatal care with good surveillance minimizes the risk of complications. Hypertensive disorders of pregnancy can result in life-threatening multisystem pathology, affecting nervous, hematological, renal, hepatic, and respiratory systems.

Preeclampsia presents with maternal features of hypertension, proteinuria, and systemic dysfunction with or without fetal syndrome. Thus, proteinuria is an objective marker and reflects the system-wide endothelial leak that characterizes the preeclampsia syndrome.

There has been an alarming 30% increase in incidence of hypertensive disorders of pregnancy [7], which is explained by the demographics of increase in maternal age, obesity, and increase in use of assisted reproductive techniques, which alters the maternal-fetal immune response. It is also influenced by genetic predisposition, race, and ethnicity.

4. Risk factors

Numerous preconceptional and pregnancy-related risk factors are identified and classified in development of preeclampsia.

4.1 Advanced maternal age

There has been variation of maternal age of pregnancy from teenage to women who are 40 years or older, as compared with women between 20 and 29 years [8] of age, with approximately twofold increase in risk of preeclampsia. Hispanic ethnicity may be at increased risk of developing preeclampsia [9]. Women with advancing age and delayed childbirth show a substantial increase in chronic hypertension during pregnancy and are at increased risk of preeclampsia.

4.2 Genetic factors

Maternal and fetal genetic factors carry strong risk for preeclampsia, with one-third attributable to maternal genetic factors [10]. Women are twice as likely to develop the disorder if they have a family history of preeclampsia, [11] and the risk increases with multiple affected pregnancies [12], potentially carrying high-risk outcomes of placental abruption and fetal growth restriction. Women with history of preeclampsia in previous pregnancy are at increased risk in subsequent pregnancy, particularly in the early onset of preeclampsia.

Partner-related risk factors are long considered a disease of primigravida in women due to limited paternal sperm antigens exposure before conception, which suggests an immunological role in pathophysiology of preeclampsia, with its incidence approximately threefold higher as compared to parous women [13]. A significant contribution of paternal genes (in the fetus) was identified as risk, with one-fifth of the variance in liability conferred through fetal genes in preeclampsia [14].

4.3 Metabolic factors

With worldwide increase in prevalence of obesity, risk of preeclampsia escalates with increasing body mass index (BMI) [15]. A systemic review found that an increase in BMI of 5–7 Kg/m was associated with a twofold increased risk of preeclampsia; it also has strong association with insulin resistance and chronic hypertension, elevating the risk of preeclampsia [16].

Other maternal medical conditions with recognized risk factors for preeclampsia are chronic renal disease, antiphospholipid antibody syndrome, and systemic lupus erythematosus [17] and pregnancy-related conditions with increased placental mass, including multiple fetal gestation and hydatidiform mole, are associated with higher rates of preeclampsia as well [18].

Associated metabolic syndrome, chronic disorders hypertension, preexisting diabetes, and renal diseases that cause endothelial injury are risk factors for preeclampsia. This explains the similar tendency of endothelial dysfunction and common factor for association of preeclampsia with increased future cardiovascular diseases [19].

4.4 Behavioral factors

Cigarette smoking during pregnancy decreases the risk of preeclampsia [20] by 30–40% as compared to women who do not smoke although biological mechanism remains unknown but probable mechanism may include nicotine inhibition of thromboxane A2 synthesis [21], simulation of nitric oxide release, or combination of both.

4.5 Recreational physical activity

Physical activity during pregnancy is associated with decreased risk for preeclampsia in non-obese women [22]. This occurs by decreasing oxidative stress, enhancing endothelial function, and modulating the immune and inflammatory response.

5. Evtiology

The exact cause of initiation and progress of the disease process is not known, with placenta being the focus in pathogenesis.

Following theories have been proposed to explain mechanics causing preeclampsia.

- Abnormal placentation with failure of trophoblast invasion of uterine vessels.
- Immunological intolerance between maternal, paternal (placental), and fetal tissues.
- Vascular endothelial damage.
- Genetic-inherited predisposition and polygenic disorders.

5.1 Abnormal placentation

In physiological pregnancy, embryo-derived endovascular cytotrophoblast invades the decidual (10–12 weeks) and myometrial (16–18 weeks) segment of spiral arterioles of uteroplacental bed, replacing endothelial lining [23] and causing remodeling of vascular smooth muscles and inner elastic lamina (**Figure 1**). These physiological changes lead the maternal spiral arterioles to distend the luminal diameter fourfold, resulting in creation of tortuous and funnel-shaped flaccid [23] tubes that provide a low-resistance, low-pressure, high-capacitance, high-flow pathway into intervillous space, which gets further remodeled and unresponsive to vasoactive stimuli. These alterations in maternal vasculature ensure adequate blood flow to nourish the growing fetus and placenta.

In preeclampsia, endovascular cytotrophoblast invasion may be incomplete [24] and only the decidual vessels undergo change, while the deeper myometrial arterioles do not lose their endothelial lining and musculoelastic tissue, resulting in narrowing of maternal spiral arterioles (**Figure 1**), thus impairing placental blood flow and remaining hyperresponsive to vasomotor stimuli. Inadequate spiral arteriolar remodeling leads to narrowing of maternal vessels and relative placental ischemia.

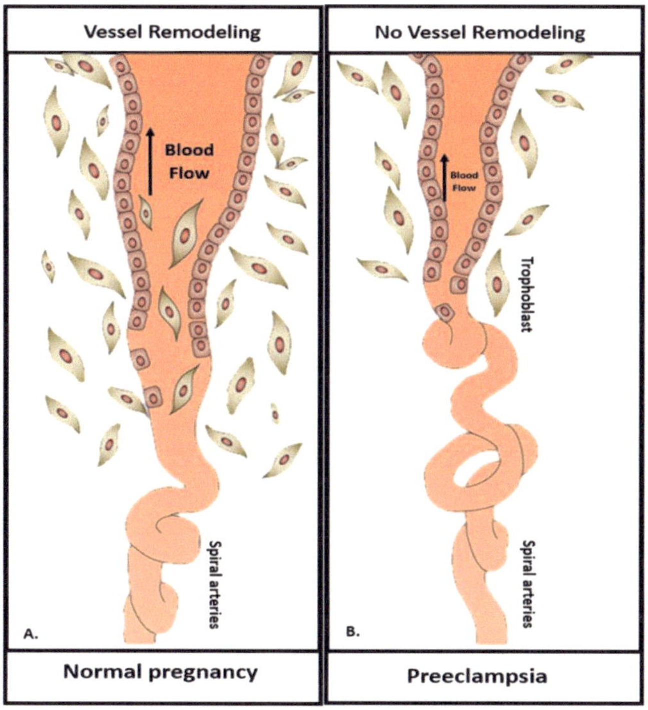

Figure 1.
A-Normal pregnancy uterine spiral arteries are wide open and remodeled by endovascular trophoblast, thereby increasing blood flow B-Preeclampsia women spiral arteries fail to remodel due to defective trophoblast invasion.

The severity of the disease correlates with the magnitude of defective trophoblastic invasion [25]. Atherosclerotic changes in maternal radial arteries that supply decidua are observed in preeclampsia. Decidual vasculopathy lesions have high association in preeclampsia with placental insufficiency, including intrauterine growth restriction and small for gestational age [26]. These changes correspond to symptomatic second stage of the preeclampsia syndrome with systemic inflammatory response [27].

In association with defective remodeling of uteroplacental vasculature, there may be presence of agonistic autoantibodies to the angiotensin receptor-1 (AT1) [28]. These autoantibodies activate AT1 receptors, endothelial cells, and vascular smooth muscle cells [29]. The autoantibodies appear to block trophoblastic invasion and may induce the production of reactive oxygen species that plays a significant role in the pathogenesis of preeclampsia at several different stages [29].

5.2 Immunological factors

Maternal immune tolerance to parentally derived placental and fetal antigens is lost at maternal-placental interface, which is suggestive of acute graft rejection. The abnormal uteroplacental development is not clearly understood but is likely due to complex interaction of immunologic, vascular, environmental, and genetic factors. The theory of immune maladaptation may play a central role in predisposition to abnormal placentation and subsequent preeclampsia, suggesting that long-term exposure to paternal antigens in sperm is protective.

In preeclamptic women, extravillous trophoblast in early pregnancy expresses reduced amounts of immunosuppressive non-classic human leukocyte antigen G (HLA G). These changes contribute to defective placental vascularization in stage 1 of preeclampsia syndrome [30].

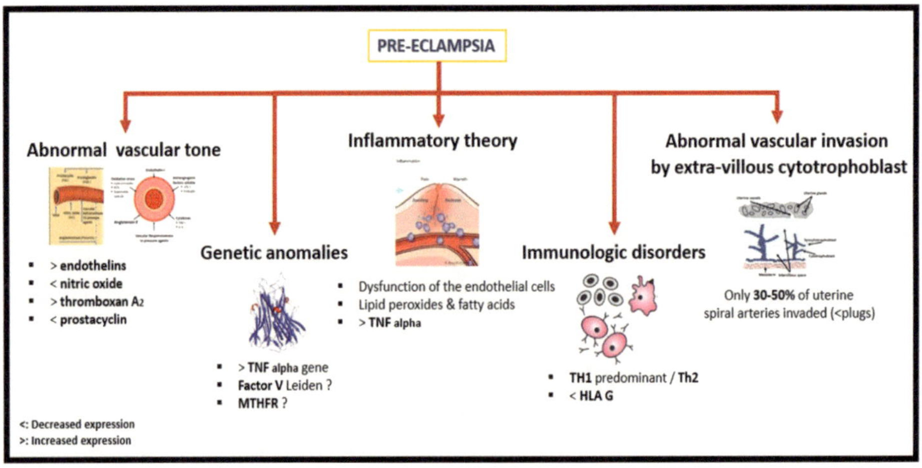

Figure 2.
Etiology of preeclampsia.

Excess macrophages in the decidua are associated with impaired trophoblast invasion and impaired placentation, signifying excess inflammation. NK cells interact with fetal trophoblast cell markers *via* killer immunoglobulin receptors (KIR) to influence trophoblastic invasion. Specific genotypic combinations of maternal KIR and trophoblastic human leukocyte antigen C (HLA-C) may increase the risk for preeclampsia. Systemic review of 22 studies examining association between HLA type and risk of preeclampsia suggests that HLA-DR correlates with preeclampsia, but it is unclear if this or any other HLA genotype is casually related to preeclampsia risk; further large sample size studies are called to examine maternal-fetal HLA combinations and risk of preeclampsia [30].

Etiology of preeclampsia is summarized in **Figure 2**.

6. Pathogenesis

6.1 Endothelial activation or dysfunction causing vasospasm

Inflammatory changes are said to be a continuation of stage 1 alternation. Placental factors are released in response to ischemia, and a cascade of events is provoked in response to antiangiogenic and metabolic factors and other inflammatory leukocyte mediators, commonly called endothelial cell activation or dysfunction. Systemic endothelial cell injury with intense vasospasm is from imbalance of vasodilators (PGI, NO), vasoconstrictors (Angiotensin-II, Thromboxane A2, and Endothelin-II), oxidative stress, and inflammatory mediators (**Figure 3**). Vasospasm exerts a damaging effect on blood vessels and causes endothelial cells to contract and, together with hypoxia, leads to hemorrhage, necrosis, and compromised end-organ function.

In preeclampsia, inflammatory mediators contributed by systemic oxidative stress are tumor necrosis factor [31] alpha (TNF-Alpha) and interleukins that in turn lead to formation of lipid peroxidases [32], producing toxic radicals that injure systemic vascular endothelial cells.

Mechanisms are precisely understood but proposed theory discussed are as follows:

- Increase in circulatory pressor substances.

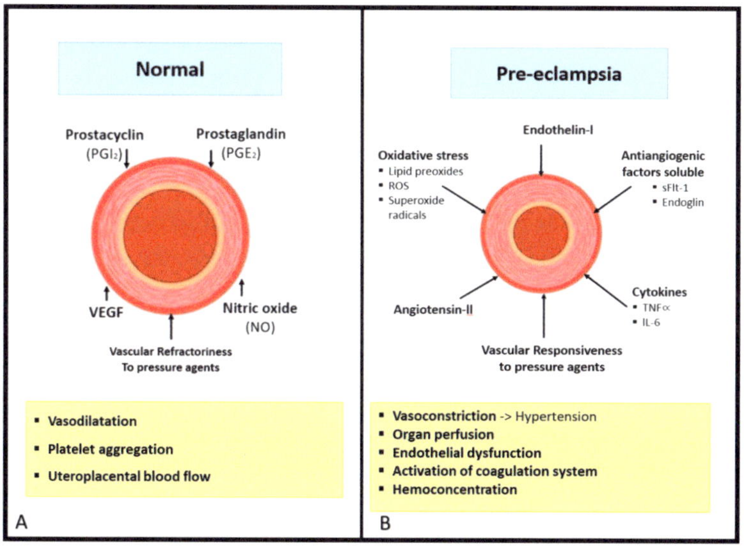

Figure 3.
A: In normal pregnancy. B: Vasoconstriction in preeclampsia.

- Increased sensitivity of the vascular system to normally circulating pressor substance.
- First-time exposure to chorionic villi.
- Superabundance of chorionic villi, exposed as with multifetal gestation or hydatidiform mole.
- Have preexisting vascular diseases associated with endothelial cell activation or inflammation such as diabetes, obesity, cardiovascular or renal, immunological disorders, or hereditary influences.
    - Genetically predisposed to hypertension developing during pregnancy.
    - Imbalance of angiogenic and antiangiogenic proteins.

6.2 Endothelial cell injury

Injury to systemic endothelial cell is crucial in pathogenesis of preeclampsia and likely secretes placental protein factors into maternal circulation, which provokes activation and dysfunction of systemic vascular endothelium, producing less nitric oxide contributing to vasoconstriction, and promotes coagulation and greater sensitivity to vasopressors.

6.3 Increased pressor responses

Normal pregnant women develop blunted vascular pressor response selectively to pressor agent angiotensin II, mediated by synthesis of endothelial prostaglandin and nitric oxide, which is a potent vasodilator. Following preeclampsia, angiotensinase activity is depressed, and the presence of autoantibodies to angiotensin AT1 receptor increases the vascular sensitivity to pressor agent angiotensin-II (**Figure 4**).

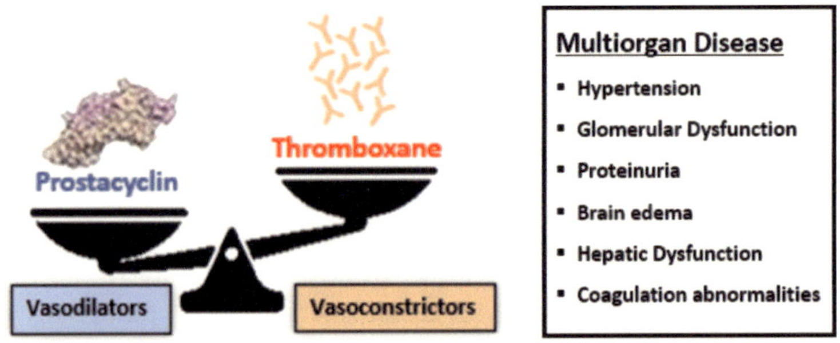

Figure 4.
Imbalance of increased thromboxane and decreased prostacyclin in preeclampsia.

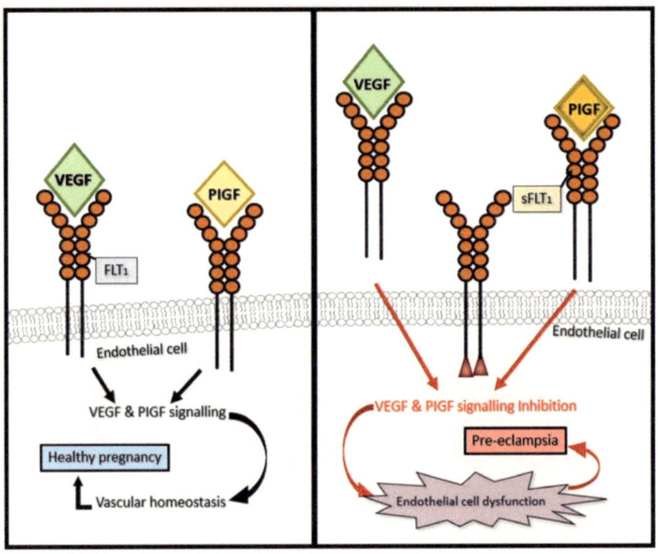

Figure 5.
Normal pregnancy: signaling of vascular hemostasias is maintained by physiological level of Vascular endothelial growth factor (VEGF) and Transforming growth factor (TGF). (B) In preeclampsia: excess secretion of Sflt1 (soluble fms- like tyrosine kinase) and sENG (soluble endoglin protein) inhibits VEGF (Vascular endothelial growth factor) and TGF (transforming growth factor) signaling of vasculature.

6.4 Angiogenic and antiangiogenic proteins

There is an imbalance of proangiogenic (VEGF) [33] and antiangiogenic (soluble fms-like tyrosine kinase sFlt-I) proteins in placental vascular bed. Soluble fms-like tyrosine kinase 1 (sFlt-1) has a receptor for VEGF (**Figure 5**).

With the progress of pregnancy, the placenta becomes relatively hypoxic at uteroplacental interface and results in an overexpression and release of placentally derived antiangiogenic peptide factors from the trophoblastic tissue, including sFlt-1 and soluble endoglin protein (sEng) into the maternal circulation, which appears to be important in pathogenesis of preeclampsia and remains the underlying theory [34]. Endothelin-I is synthesized by endothelial cells and is a potent vasoconstrictor causing hypertension (**Figure 5**).

In preeclampsia, sFlt-1 is a soluble antiangiogenic protein that is elevated, which binds and inactivates or reduces biological activity of free-circulating proangiogenic proteins, vascular endothelial growth factor (VEGF), and placental growth factor (PIGF), causing endothelial dysfunction [35].

7. Systemic organ dysfunction and complications

Severe manifestations of preeclampsia occur in all body systems because of widespread endothelial dysfunction, making diagnosis difficult due to similar clinical presentation despite complex differences in their underlying pathophysiology and prognosis.

Numerous factors combine to exert vasoactive effects in preeclampsia [36], causing resistance to blood flow and accounts for the development of arterial hypertension. Systemic organ dysfunction is explained in **Figure 6**.

7.1 Central nervous system dysfunction

Two marked cerebral pathologies are gross hemorrhage and ischemia, with other common variable lesions noted are edema, hyperemia, and thrombosis.

Manifestations of the central nervous system are severe headache, hyperexcitability, hyperreflexia, and coma attributable to hypoxia. Reversible vasogenic cerebral edema occurs commonly due to endothelial dysfunction of the brain in preeclampsia and eclampsia. Failure of autoregulation with reduced global cerebral blood flow and hyperperfusion commonly occurs in posterior circulation, such that the changes in the brain of patients with preeclampsia/eclampsia result in posterior reversible leukoencephalopathy syndrome (PRES) [37].

Intense ocular arteriolar constriction may cause visual disturbances, and may include blurred vision, scotoma, amaurosis [38], and retinal detachment (**Figure 7**).

Airway: In normal healthy pregnancy, the internal diameter of the trachea is reduced because of mucosal capillary engorgement, which can be exaggerated with narrowing of upper airway, resulting in pharyngolaryngeal edema, and subglottic edema with signs of airway obstructions such as dysphonia, hoarseness, snoring, stridor, and hypoxemia; these changes may compromise visualization of airway landmarks during direct laryngoscopy making intubation difficult [39].

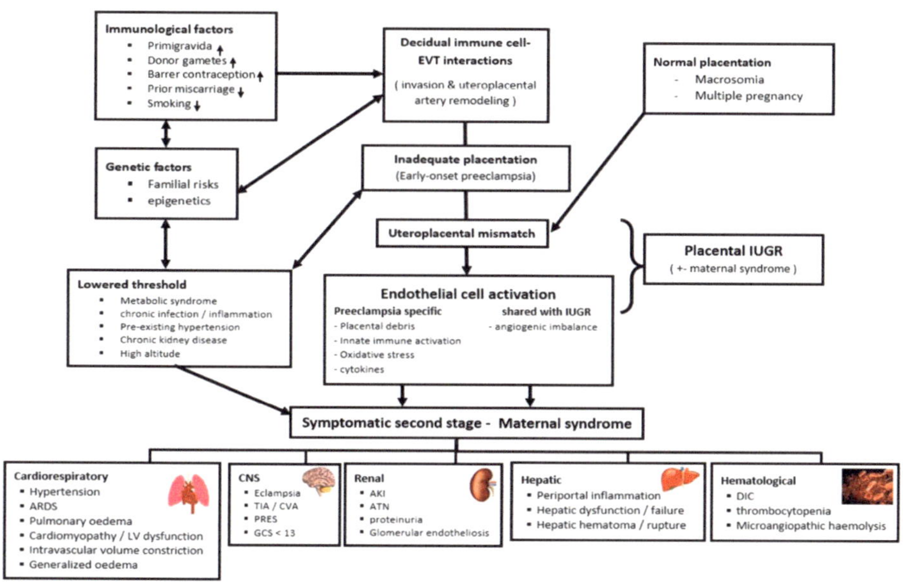

Figure 6.
Etiopathogenesis of preeclampsia.

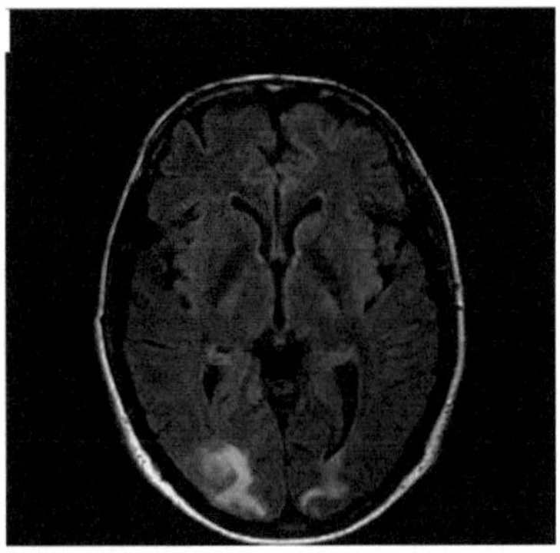

Figure 7.
PRES syndrome.

7.2 Respiratory system dysfunction

Pulmonary edema occurs in approximately 3% of preeclamptic women [40]. It is relatively infrequent in young healthy women than multiparous women. Decreased colloid osmotic pressure, in combination with increased permeability and the loss of intravascular fluid and protein into the interstitium, increases the risk for pulmonary edema [41]. Endothelial activations lead to extravasation of intravascular fluid into the extracellular space and, importantly, into the lungs. Excess intravenous fluid administration is an important risk factor for pulmonary edema in preeclampsia patients [42].

7.3 Cardiovascular system dysfunction

Common cardiovascular disturbances in preeclampsia syndrome are increased afterload caused by hypertension and reduced preload by pathologically diminished volume expansion during pregnancy.

Preeclampsia is a hyperdynamic state with increased vascular tone and increased sensitivity to vasoconstrictor, resulting in clinical manifestation of hypertension, vasospasm, and end-organ ischemia [43]. Hemodynamic response to circulatory catecholamine is exaggerated and characterized by severe vasospasm. Typically, blood pressure and systemic vascular resistance are elevated.

The majority of preeclamptic women show increased cardiac output [44], mild-to-moderate increased systemic vascular resistance [45], and hyperdynamic left ventricular function.

In summary, aggressive fluid administration in severe preeclampsia substantially elevates left-sided filling pressures and cardiac output to hyperdynamic levels. This elevates pulmonary capillary wedge pressure, causing pulmonary edema despite normal ventricular function.

7.4 Hematologic system dysfunction

Increase in blood volume is not evident in severe preeclampsia due to vasospastic state that follows endothelial activation and worsens with increased vascular permeability, and leakage of plasma into the interstitial space, resulting in increased hemoconcentration and hematocrit values that signify preeclampsia. These women with severe hemoconcentration are unduly sensitive to blood loss at delivery than normal [45].

7.5 Maternal thrombocytopenia

Thrombocytopenia is the most common hematologic disorder with platelet count of less than 100,000/mm^3 in severe preeclampsia disease or HELLP (hemolysis elevated liver function low platelets) syndrome [46] that creates a hypocoagulable state correlating with the severity of the disease process.

In preeclampsia [47], platelets are activated, subsequent degranulation accounting for decrease in platelet function, and aggregation appears to account for the decrease in platelet count.

HELLP syndrome: It is characterized by hemolysis, elevated levels of liver enzymes, and low platelet count. It is associated with increased rates of maternal and perinatal morbidity. Weinstein coined the acronym HELLP. Women who do not reveal one or more of the clinical features is called partial HELLP syndrome [48].

Clinical presentation of maternal signs and symptoms vary from right upper quadrant or epigastric pain, nausea and vomiting, headache, hypertension, and proteinuria, and 12–18% of women may be normotensive and 13% may be without proteinuria. Clinical management has to prioritize maternal stability, particularly, hypertension and Coagulation abnormalities, and assess the fetal condition *via* FHR monitoring. Risk of postpartum hemorrhage is significantly increased in HELLP patients [48].

7.6 Hemolysis

Severe preeclampsia is frequently accompanied by microangiopathic hemolysis that manifests as elevated lactate dehydrogenase, reduced haptoglobin levels, hemolytic anemia, and abnormal peripheral blood smear with schistocytes, spherocytes, and reticulocytosis [49].

7.7 Coagulation changes

Disseminated intravascular coagulation is a syndrome secondary to microthrombi formation in severe preeclampsia with liver derangement [50]. Activation of coagulation system is marked by consumptions of procoagulants, increased levels of fibrin degradation products, and end-organ dysfunction. In advanced stages of DIC (disseminated intravascular coagulation), it may cause spontaneous hemorrhage, intrauterine fetal demise, placental abruption, or postpartum hemorrhage.

7.8 Endocrine and hormonal alternations

Plasma levels of renin, angiotensin I & II, aldosterone, deoxycorticosterone, and atrial natriuretic peptide (ANP) are substantially increased during normal pregnancy, which is further enhanced in preeclampsia women.

7.9 Fluid and electrolyte alterations

Extracellular fluid manifests as edema with pathological fluid retention in women with severe preeclampsia due to endothelial injury. In addition to generalized edema and proteinuria, these women have reduced plasma oncotic pressure, which creates a filtration imbalance and further displaces intravascular fluid into the surrounding interstitium, creating intravascular dehydration and extravascular overhydration. Electrolyte concentration does not differ grossly in preeclampsia patients.

7.10 Renal dysfunction

Defining component of preeclampsia is proteinuria, with its renal manifestations of persistent proteinuria, changes in glomerular filtration rate, renal blood flow, and hyperuricemia. In preeclampsia serum markers, blood urea nitrogen BUN, creatinine, and uric acid reflect a decrease in renal functions. Hyperuricemia (elevated uric acid levels) is one of the recognized early predictors of preeclampsia, with the primary mechanism of decreased renal clearance [51]. High level of serum uric acid correlates with the severity of the disease. Glomerular endotheliosis is the main feature of the preeclamptic kidney defined by endothelial swelling and glomerular capillary narrowing.

Oliguria is a probable late manifestation and parallels the severity of preeclampsia. Persistent oliguria (< 500-mL urine output in 24 hours) requires immediate attention for evaluation of intravascular volume status.

Major pathological process of acute renal failure in preeclampsia (83–90%) is from prerenal and intrarenal pathology (most commonly acute tubular necrosis), which resolves completely after delivery.

7.11 Hepatic dysfunction

Reduced blood flow to the liver may lead to periportal necrosis and are at risk of periportal hemorrhage, fibrin deposit, subcapsular bleeding, and hepatic rupture.

Hepatic involvement frequently presents as right upper quadrant or epigastric pain and accounts for 32% maternal mortality rate [50].

Rupture of a subcapsular hematoma of the liver is a life-threatening complication that can manifest as abdominal pain, which worsens over time and becomes localized to the epigastric area or right upper quadrant associated with nausea, vomiting, and headache. Alarming hypotension and shock develop with enlarged and tender liver. Diagnosis of liver subcapsular hematoma is confirmed by ultrasonography, computerized tomography (CT), or magnetic resonant imaging (MRI). The most common cause of death is coagulopathy. Conservative management is recommended for subcapsular hematoma or intraparenchymal hemorrhage without capsular rupture in stable women with an important component to avoid all potential trauma to the liver.

7.12 Uteroplacental malperfusion

Uteroplacental perfusion can be impaired in pregnancies complicated by preeclampsia with increased downstream resistance in the uteroplacental bed, decreased diastolic flow velocity, and increased systolic-diastolic flow velocity ratio [51]. Reduced uteroplacental malperfusion is considered one of the major causes of fetal compromise (IUGR, premature birth, and perinatal death). Risk of placental abruption is increased threefold with increased perinatal morbidity and mortality in preeclampsia women [51].

8. General principles and management

- Definite treatment of preeclampsia is termination of pregnancy to prevent disease progression and reduce maternal complications and neonatal morbidity. Time of delivery is based on gestational age, severity of preeclampsia, and maternal and fetal condition.

- Birth of infant who can then thrive subsequently.
- Most patients with preeclampsia with or without severe features can be delivered vaginally. Cesarean delivery is indicated for obstetric indications.
- Fluid balance must be titrated closely to avoid excessive administration and avoid pulmonary edema.
- Expectant management of women with preeclampsia without severe features of disease process may be considered in tertiary care center setting with maternal-fetal medicine specialist (frequent laboratory monitoring, and clinical assessment of mother and fetus).
- Complete restoration of mother's health.

9. Long-term consequences

Table 1 describes long-term complications of preeclampsia syndrome.

Cardiovascular	Neurovascular	Metabolic	Renal	Central nervous system
Chronic hypertension	Stroke	Type 2 diabetes	Glomerular dysfunction	Cognitive dysfunction
Ischemic heart disease	Retinal detachment	Metabolic syndrome	Proteinuria	Retinopathy
Atherosclerosis	Diabetic retinopathy	Obesity		White-matter lesions
Cardiomyopathy		Dyslipidemia		
Thromboembolism				

Table 1.
Long-term impact of preeclampsia.

10. Conclusion

Preeclampsia is one of the hypertensive disorders of pregnancy with increased morbidity and mortality. It occurs in up to 12% of pregnancies. Advanced maternal age, genetic factors, obesity, and chronic renal impairment increase the risk of preeclampsia in pregnant patients. Abnormal placentation, immunological changes, endothelial injury and activation, and increased pressor response are the pathogenesis of preeclampsia.

Due to these generalized endothelial changes, the preeclampsia patients develop multiple organ dysfunction, including PRES (posterior reversible encephalopathy) syndrome, pulmonary edema, HELLP syndrome, acute kidney injury, and uteroplacental insufficiencies.

Management of preeclampsia is supportive therapy, blood pressure control, and seizures prevention and delivery of the fetus. Long-term effects of preeclampsia are chronic hypertension, stroke, and chronic kidney disease.

Author details

Nissar Shaikh[1*], Seema Nahid[2], Firdous Ummunnisa[3], Ifrah Fatima[4], Mohamad Hilani[4], Asma Gul[4], A. Al Basha[4], W. Yahia[2], F. Al Hail[4], H. Elfil[1], E. Abdalla[1], M.M. Nainthramveetil[2], M.A Imraan[2], Muhammad Zubair[2], Sibghatulla Khan[2], N. Korichi[4], S. Alkhawaga[4], H. Ismail[4], S. Yaqoob[4] and Mashael Abdulrahman M.S. Al Khelaifi[4]

1 Surgical Intensive Care Unit: Hamad Medical Corporation, Doha, Qatar

2 Department of Anesthesia/ICU and Perioperative Medicine: Hamad Medical Corporation, Doha, Qatar

3 Dr. Halima Al Tamimi, Obstetrics and Gynaecology Centre, Doha, Qatar

4 Women Wellness and Research Center: Hamad Medical Corporation, Doha, Qatar

*Address all correspondence to: nissatfirdous99@gmail.com

References

[1] Ananth CV, Keyes KM, Wapner RJ. Pre-eclampsia rates in the United States 1980-2010: Age-period-cohort analysis. BMJ. 2013;**347**:6564.2

[2] Hutcheon JA, Lisonkova S, Joseph KS. Epidemiology of pre-eclampsia and the other hypertensive disorders of pregnancy. Best Practice & Research. Clinical Obstetrics & Gynaecology. 2011;**25**:391-403

[3] Brown MA, Lindheimer MD, de Swiet M, et al. The classification and diagnosis of the hypertensive disorders of pregnancy: Statement from the International Society for the Study of Hypertension in Pregnancy (ISSHP). Hypertension in Pregnancy. 2001; **20**:IX-XIV

[4] Say L, Chou D, Gemmill A, et al. Global causes of maternal death: A WHO systematic analysis. The Lancet Global Health. 2014;**2**(6):e323-e333

[5] Hogan MC, Foreman KJ, Naghavi M, Ahn SY, Wang M, Makela SM, et al. Maternal mortality for 181 countries, 1980-2008: A systematic analysis of progress towards Millennium Development Goal 5. Lancet. 2010; **375**:1609-1623

[6] Gant NF, Daley GL, Chand S, et al. A study of angiotensin II pressor response throughout primigravid pregnancy. The Journal of Clinical Investigation. 1973; **52**:2682-2689

[7] Kuklina EV, Ayala C, Callaghan WM. Hypertensive disorders and severe obstetric morbidity in the United States. Obstetrics and Gynecology. 2009; **113**:1299-1306

[8] Bianco A, Stone J, Lynch L, et al. Pregnancy outcome at age 40and older. Obstetrics and Gynecology. 1996; **87**:917-922

[9] Cnattingius S, Reilly M, Pawitan Y, Lichtenstein P. Maternal and fetal genetic factors account for most of familial aggregation of Preeclampsia: A population-based Swedish cohort study. American Journal of Medical Genetics. Part A. 2004;**130A**:365-371

[10] Mogren I, Hogberg U, Winkvist A, Stenlund H. Familial occurrence of preeclampsia. Epidemiology. 1999; **10**:518-522

[11] Hernandez-Diaz S, Toh S, Cnattingius S. Risk of pre-eclampsia in first and subsequent pregnancies: Prospective cohort study. BMJ. 2009; **338**:b2255

[12] Duckitt K, Harrington D. Risk factors for pre-eclampsia at antenatal booking: Systematic review of controlled studies. BMJ. 2005;**330**:565

[13] O'Brien TE, Ray JG, Chan WS. Maternal body mass index and the risk of preeclampsia: A systematic overview. Epidemiology. 2003;**14**:368-374

[14] Nevis IF, Reitsma A, Dominic A, et al. Pregnancy outcomes in women with chronic kidney disease: A systematic review. Clinical Journal of the American Society of Nephrology. 2011;**6**:2587-2598

[15] Koga K, Osuga Y, Tajima T, et al. Elevated serum soluble fms-like tyrosine kinase 1 (sFlt1) level in women with hydatidiform mole. Fertility and Sterility. 2010;**94**:305-308

[16] Wallis AB, Saftlas AF, Hsia J, Atrash HK. Secular trends in the rates of preeclampsia, eclampsia, and gestational hypertension. American Journal of Hypertension. 2008; **21**:521-526

[17] Conde-Agudelo A, Althabe F, Belizan JM, Kafury-Goeta AC. Cigarette smoking during pregnancy and risk of

preeclampsia: A systematic review. American Journal of Obstetrics and Gynecology. 1999;**181**:1026-1035

[18] Funai EF, Friedlander Y, Paltiel O, et al. Long-term mortality after preeclampsia. Epidemiology. 2005; **16**:206-215

[19] Sorensen TK, Williams MA, Lee IM, et al. Recreational physical activity during pregnancy and risk of preeclampsia. Hypertension. 2003; **41**:1273-1280

[20] Powe CE, Levine RJ, Karumanchi SA. Preeclampsia, a disease of the maternal endothelium: The role of antiangiogenic factors and implications for later cardiovascular disease. Circulation. 2011;**123**:2856-2869

[21] Brosens I, Robertson WB, Dixon HG. The physiological response of the vessels of the placental bed to normal pregnancy. The Journal of Pathology and Bacteriology. 1967; **93**:569-579

[22] Zhou Y, Damsky CH, Fisher SJ. Preeclampsia is associated with failure of human cytotrophoblasts to mimic a vascular adhesion phenotype. The Journal of Clinical Investigation. 1997; **99**(9):2152

[23] Madazli R, Budak E, Calay Z, et al. Correlation between placental bed biopsy findings, vascular cell adhesion molecule and fibronectin levels in preeclampsia. BJOG. 2000;**107**:514

[24] Hecht JL, Zsengeller ZK, Spiel M, Karumanchi SA, Rosen S. Revisiting decidual vasculopathy. Placenta. 2016;**42**:37-43. DOI: 10.1016/j.placenta.2016.04.006

[25] Lee SM, Romero R, Lee YJ, et al. Systemic inflammatory stimulation by microparticles derived from hypoxic trophoblast as a model for inflammatory response in preeclampsia. American Journal of Obstetrics and Gynecology. 2012;**207**(4):337.e1

[26] Wallukat G, Homuth V, Fischer T, et al. Patients with preeclampsia develop agonistic autoantibodies against the angiotensin AT1 receptor. The Journal of Clinical Investigation. 1999;**103**:945-952

[27] Xia Y, Wen H, Bobst S, et al. Maternal autoantibodies from preeclamptic patients activate angiotensin receptors on human trophoblast cells. Journal of the Society for Gynecologic Investigation. 2003;**10**:82-93

[28] Saftlas AF, Beydoun H, Triche E. Immunogenetic determinants of preeclampsia and related pregnancy disorders: A systematic review. Obstetrics and Gynecology. 2005; **106**:162-172

[29] Many A, Hubel CA, Fisher SJ, Roberts JM, Zhou Y. Invasive cytotrophoblasts manifest evidence of oxidative stress in preeclampsia. The American Journal of Pathology. 2000; **156**:321-331

[30] Manten GT, van der Hoek YY, Marko Sikkema J, et al. The role of lipoprotein (a) in pregnancies complicated by pre-eclampsia. Medical Hypotheses. 2005;**64**:162-169

[31] Redman CW, Sargent IL. Latest advances in understanding preeclampsia. Science. 2005; **308**:1592-1594

[32] Smith GN, Walker M, Tessier JL, Millar KG. Increased incidence of preeclampsia in women conceiving by intrauterine insemination with donor versus partner sperm for treatment of primary infertility. American Journal of Obstetrics and Gynecology. 1997; **177**(2):455-458

[33] Kendall RL, Thomas KA. Inhibition of vascular endothelial cell growth

factor activity by an endogenously encoded soluble receptor. Proceedings of the National Academy of Sciences USA. 1993;**90**:10705-10709

[34] Oudejans CB, van Dijk M, Oosterkamp M, et al. Genetics of preeclampsia: Paradigm shifts. Human Genetics. 2007;**120**:607-612

[35] Davison JM, Dunlop W. Renal hemodynamics and tubular function normal human pregnancy. Kidney International. 1980;**18**:152-161

[36] Liman TG, Bohner G, Heuschmann PU, et al. Clinical and radiological differences in posterior reversible encephalopathy syndrome between patients with preeclampsia-eclampsia and other predisposing diseases. European Journal of Neurology. 2012;**19**:935-943

[37] Munnur U, de Boisblanc B, Suresh MS. Airway problems in pregnancy. Critical Care Medicine. 2005;**33** Suppl. 10:S259-S268

[38] Sibai BM, Mabie BC, Harvey CJ, Gonzalez AR. Pulmonary edema in severe preeclampsia-eclampsia: Analysis of thirty-seven consecutive cases. American Journal of Obstetrics and Gynecology. 1987;**156**:1174-1179

[39] Benedetti TJ, Kates R, Williams V. Hemodynamic observations in severe preeclampsia complicated by pulmonary edema. American Journal of Obstetrics and Gynecology. 1985; **152**:330-334

[40] Thornton CE, von Dadelszen P, Makris A, et al. Acute pulmonary oedema as a complication of hypertension during pregnancy. Hypertension in Pregnancy. 2011; **30**:169-179

[41] Roberts JM, Cooper DW. Pathogenesis and genetics of preeclampsia. Lancet. 2001;**357**:53-56

[42] Kobayashi T, Tokunaga N, Isoda H, et al. Vasospasms are characteristic in cases with eclampsia/preeclampsia and HELLP syndrome: Proposal of an angiospastic syndrome of pregnancy. Seminars in Thrombosis and Hemostasis. 2001;**27**:131-135

[43] Zeeman GG, Cunningham FG, Pritchard JA. The magnitude of hemoconcentration with eclampsia. Hypertension in Pregnancy. 2009; **28**(2):127

[44] Sibai B, Dekker G, Kupferminc M. Pre-eclampsia. Lancet. 2005; **365**:785-799

[45] Harlow FH, Brown MA, Brighton TA, et al. Platelet activation in the hypertensive disorders of pregnancy. American Journal of Obstetrics and Gynecology. 2002;**187**:688-695

[46] Thachil J, Toh CH. Disseminated intravascular coagulation in obstetric disorders and its acute haematological management. Blood Reviews. 2009; **23**:167-176

[47] Cunningham FG, Lowe T, Guss S, et al. Erythrocyte morphology in women with severe preeclampsia and eclampsia. American Journal of Obstetrics and Gynecology. 1985; **153**:358

[48] Weinstein L. Syndrome of hemolysis, elevated liver enzymes, and low platelet count: A severe consequence of hypertension in pregnancy. American Journal of Obstetrics and Gynecology. 1982;**142**:159-167

[49] Siemens J, Bogert L. The uric acid content of maternal and fetal blood. The Journal of Biological Chemistry. 1917;**32**:63-67

[50] Rinehart BK, Terrone DA, Magann EF, et al. Preeclampsia associated hepatic hemorrhage and rupture: Mode of management related

to maternal and perinatal outcome. Obstetrical & Gynecological Survey. 1999;**54**:196-202

[51] Trudinger BJ, Giles WB, Cook CM, et al. Fetal umbilical artery flow velocity waveforms and placental resistance: Clinical significance. BJOG. 1985; **92**:23-30

Section 5

Gestational Endothelialpathy

Chapter 5

Gestational Endotheliopathy as Trigger Disorder of Haemodynamics Pregnancy Supply

Dmytro Konkov, George Belkania, Levon Dilenyan, Victor Rud, Liana Puchalska, Alina Piskun and Larisa Klimas

Abstract

The idea for this study is based on endothelial-dependent adaptation of hemodynamic circulation in pregnancy. The optimization of the circulatory component of the cardiovascular system (CVS) during pregnancy via blood pressure (BP), especially in physiological pregnancy (PhP), is accompanied by a clear overall increase in systolic characteristics of the pumping function of the heart. This orientation in cardiac output (CO) is unambiguously manifested throughout all three trimesters as with PhP—in a prone and standing position in total according to 24 characteristics out of 24 ($P < 0.01$), while for gestational endotheliopathy (PaP)—by 18 out of 24 ($P < 0.05$) clear restructuring of the dynamic organization of the circulatory state according to the anthropophysiological ratio to the hyperkinetic state according to CO in a standing position (type III) was noted with all blood pressure (BP) regimes. If the manifestation of type III under hypotonic, normotonic, and hypertonic regimes in BP was 8, 12, and 6%, respectively, then in the case of PhP, it was 21, 36, and 50%, respectively ($P < 0.01$), and for PaP, it was 48, 66, and 76% ($P < 0.01$). Hemodynamically identified heart failure (HF) syndrome, as the earliest preclinical circulatory endothelial-dependent form, is examined as a trigger of formation of perinatal pathology corresponding to preeclampsia.

Keywords: pregnancy, gestational endotheliopathy, perinatal pathology, cardiovascular system, circulation, pumping function of heart, cardiac output, cardiac index, heart failure

1. Introduction

In early gestational age, the decidua has been extensively studied to define the spiral artery remodeling process that occurs during pregnancy. The remodeling results from a complex interaction between maternal decidual immune cells in the uterine wall and invasive trophoblasts. During remodeling the arterial muscular layer is replaced by fibrinoid material, and the arterial diameter increases 4–12-fold [1, 2]. The process of optimal trophoblast invasion is often defective in preeclampsia, particularly in early-onset preeclampsia, affecting the endothelium (gestational endotheliopathy) but not the interstitial invasion pathway; the remodeling of myometrial spiral artery segments is particularly affected. However, defective remodeling is also seen in other cases of perinatal pathology and even rarely in normal pregnancy. The resulting abnormal uteroplacental flow is associated with placental oxidative stress, probably from ischemia reperfusion injury of the placenta. It is not known why some woman with gestational endotheliopathy develop preeclampsia, while others do not [3–6].

It is important to understand that all organism mechanisms providing pregnancy depend, foremost, on the hemodynamic system and the priority role of the perfusion complex (volume–tube–pump–pressure–blood flow)—pumping function of heart. More research assures that preeclampsia is examined not so much as the first event in subsequent development for women with cardiovascular diseases [7], but rather as a special circulatory state due to not insufficient, in our view, but tense adaptation of the CVS [8–10] in women, as straight-walking creatures, in pregnancy. However, a faithful a faithful parcel in determination of relations reason-result determines the necessity of establishment of certain factor or terms, according to which such adaptations show up in the CVS in pregnancy, and also determination of hemodynamic structure of perfusion mechanisms lying in and defining the orientation of this adaptation at physiological and pathological pregnancy. Such synergy substantially impacts tension of adjusting of blood circulation on a gravitational factor, especially in the upright position. In turn, antigravity tension of the CVS affects the blood circulation of pregnant women, which is critical for maintenance and development of fetoplacental circulation of blood. The real influence of formed biophysical terms related to pregnancy shows up from the second half of pregnancy, on circulation of blood and in the lying position [10–12].

Some studies have shown an association that displays growth of circulatory tension and gestational endotheliopathy of typology alteration of dynamic organization of CVS with growth of hyperkinetic state of circulation of blood in position straight standing-type III of antropophysiological correlation (upright/lying, %), minute volume of blood (MVB), system resistance of arterial vessels, especially on circulatory responsible regions (abdominal and pelvic circulation of blood), often combining with the ischemic state, together with the increase of hemodynamically identified [13, 14] circulatory syndromes of heart failure (HF). Obtained data suggest that antigravity tension of the CVS is a circulatory basis for both early and late preeclampsia. It is thus necessary to mean that blood pressure (BP) in pregnant, to that attention is brought over its determination of the state of preeclampsia, is the external display (a result, but not reason) of adaptation changes of all difficult complex of maternal circulation of blood, especially its basic mechanisms of perfusion, in the hemodynamic fetoplacental complex and, actually, organism of pregnant. Orthostatic proteinuria, which in preeclampsia is associated with arterial high BP, reflects tension of kidney link in the adaptation of the CVS to the gravitational factor of circulation of blood and out of pregnancy [15, 16].

The aim of this study is antropophysiological analysis of the circulatory state of the CVS in PhP and pregnancy with gestational endotheliopathy as a trigger, in the development of hemodynamic supply disorder in pregnancy and perinatal pathology (PaP).

2. Materials and methods

The study was performed at the National Pirogov Memorial Medical University, Vinnytsya, Ukraine, under budget grant No. 0121 U109141. Observational clinical studies were undertaken on 114 women with physiological pregnancy (PhP) and 131 pregnant women with perinatal pathology (PaP). The former group consisted of 23 women in their first trimester, 38 women in their second trimester, and 55 women in their third trimester, whereas the latter group consisted of 20 women in their first trimester, 36 women in their second trimester, and 75 women in their third trimester. A control group was formed by 115 healthy nonpregnant women. General age of pregnant women was 17–36 years ($n = 245$); only four pregnant women were older than 30 years.

We enrolled pregnant women with gestational endotheliopathy, who were diagnosed when microalbuminuria was more than 5.0 mg/mmol (screening test) and endothelium-dependent vasodilation was less than 10% (approving test).

Multicentral description of "hemodynamic model" of the examined conditions (not pregnant and pregnant women) was made basis on antropophysiological research [6] of the circulatory state of the CVS, using the diagnostic system ANTROPOS-CAVASCREEN [17], which is an innovative diagnostic complex for analyzing the performance of various blood circulation sections using noninvasive methods (thoracal and regional tetrapolar rheography, electrocardiography, BP measurement, electrometrial features of skin).

According to basic criteria and syndromal analysis of multicentral complex of hemodynamic characteristics [18–21] of the "hemodynamic model" of providing of pregnancy [22] was held special antropophysiological analysis of showing up (part in % on a selection) of the different modes is conducted on middle blood pressure (BPm)—hypo-, normo- and hypertensive on positions of body upright and lying. For determining raised and lowered BPm, we used general normative descriptions of systolic BP (<140 and > 90 mmHg) and diastolic BP (<90 and > 60 mmHg). According to our special diagnostic scale, [23] group normative descriptions for BPm = BPd + 0.32*(BPs-BPd) in the lying position were well associated with the accepted diagnostic criteria; for women up to age 35 years, BPm was 79–105 mmHg. In standing position, there have been used connected to antropophysiological characteristics correlations of BPm to its criteria in position lying (in %), that allowed to identify the adaptive orientation of adjusting on the mode of BP in position upright, in that influence of gravitational (hydrostatical) factor of circulation of blood maximally impact circulatory state of the CVS. According to used criterion and by syndromal analysis [24, 25], criteria of raised and lowered BP were identified, as well as normotensive state.

With the examined modes for BP was analyzed expression of circulatory syndromes of HF at them hemodynamically identified by diagnostic algorithm worked out by us [26], as a system estimation of pumping function of heart (PFH) in the circulatory state of the CVS. PFH additionally was estimated by trimester measuring of cardiac output (CO, ml) and cardiac index on body weight (CI, ml/kg) separately in standing and lying positions. By antropophysiological ratio of CO upright/lying (APR, %) typological description of dynamic organization of the circulatory state of the CVS was made [27]. The last was presented by three types of blood circulation: type I or hypokinetic state, with the decrease of BP in standing position (93% and less) comparing to it's size in a prone position; type II or eukinetic state, with BP of 94-106% from standing to lying position; and type III or hyperkinetic state, with increase of BP up to 107% or more in the upright position.

For the integral estimation of the analyzed condition of the CVS we additionally used system characteristics, including syndrome of greater biological age (aging, age-related depreciation) and syndrome of hemodynamic risk [5, 17] on the index of hemodynamic non-optimality (IHU > 30%), as well as regional and system estimation of syndrome of resistance (vasoconstrictions) of the arterial vessels of the head, lungs, stomach, pelvis, femur, and calf [13, 14], and increases of the systolic post-loading (post+) on the left (LV) and right (RV) ventricles of the heart.

For statistical description of obtained data methods of variation and non-parametric analysis were used with Microsoft Excel 2010. Evaluation was performed by variations of criteria of student, non-parametric to the criteria of signs and rule of specificity of predominating of bigger part of a selection or compared sub-groups (part) in selections of "control-pregnant" and "physiological pregnancy vs pathological pregnancy" [28] with the accepted level of probability no less than 95%.

3. Results and discussion

Data on mBP for nonpregnant (control) and pregnant women were analyzed on general and actual selections on the BP mode. General selections were formed on correlation of BP "upright or lying." Decreased BP "upright or lying" is hypotonic mode ("−" marks), increased BP "upright or lying" is hypertensive mode (it marks "+"), and accordance of BP to normative limits "lying and upright" is the normotonic state ("0" marks). The actual modes were formed on the real combination of the modes for BP upright/lying with corresponding marks (−0+/−0+) (see **Figures 1** and **2**). It should be noted that in the normotonic mode—general ("0") and to the variants actual (0/−+) normative description of changes of BP upright there is however a primary increase of pressure, pressure orientation in adjusting of CVS in position upright.

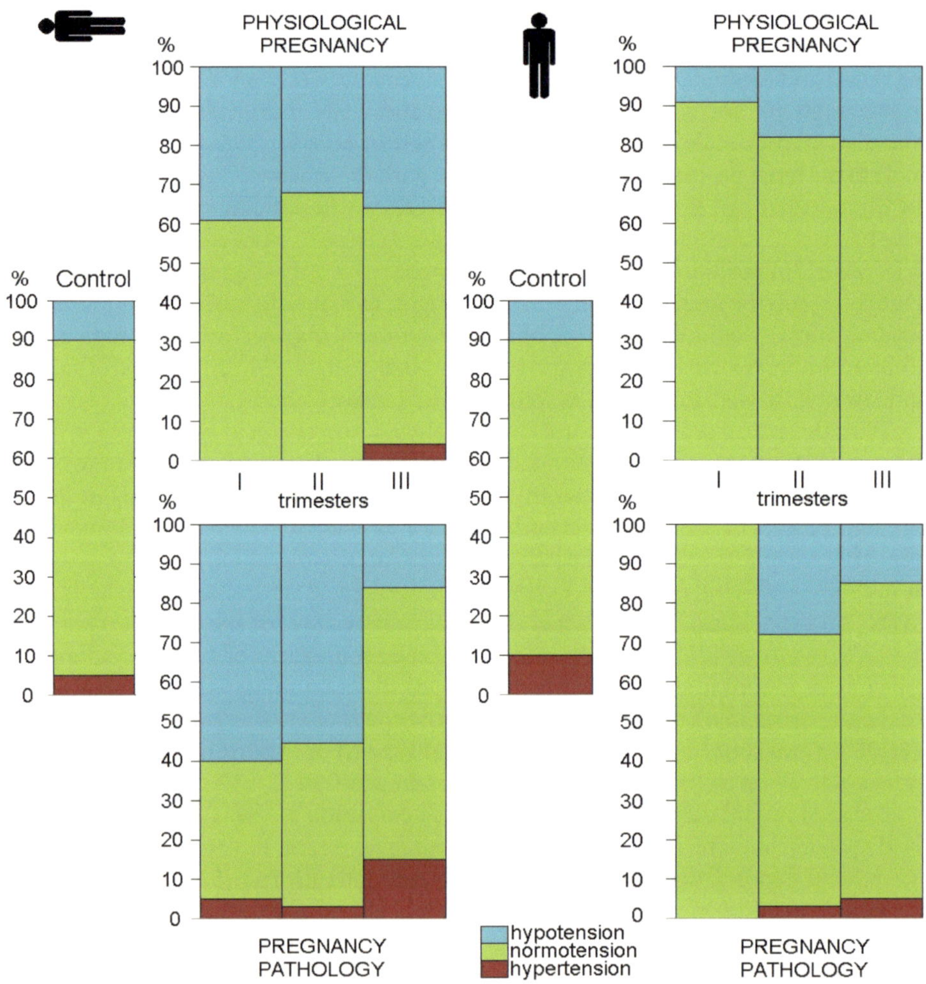

Figure 1.
Distribution of stake of people (in %) with the general modes of cardiovascular system according to BP (normotonic—Upright and lying, high blood pressure and hypotension—Upright or lying) for women of reproductive age (control) and in the first, second, and third trimesters of PhP and PaP.

It is necessary to mean that in position upright taking into account expression of the hypertensive state totally with a normative increase of BP the stake of the states of CVS of pressor orientation for women arrives at 90–92%, demonstrating actuality of the tense of pressor adjustment in adaptation of CVS to the gravitational

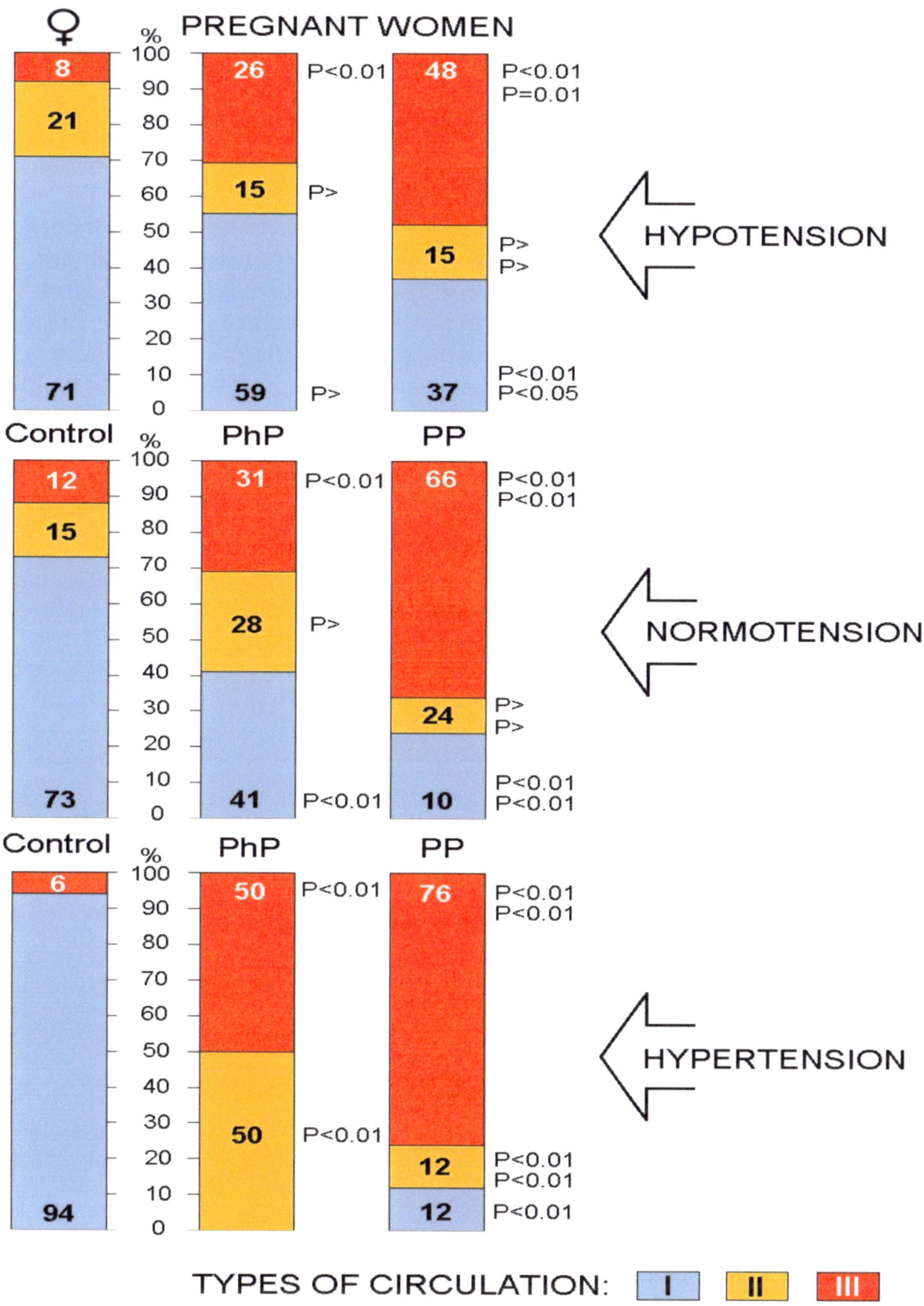

Figure 2.
Distribution of types of circulation (numbers on a diagram are a stake in % on a selection) in antropophysiological ratio of cardiac output (CO) upright/lying—Hypokinetic (I), eukinetic (II), and hyperkinetic (III) at the general modes of BP (hypotension, normotension, hypertension) of the circulatory state of CVS for nonpregnant women (control), PhP, and PaP. Authenticity of distinction (D) on the types of circulation is brought between control and PhP, by control and PaP (first row), and between PhP and PaP (second row).

(hydrostatical) factor of circulation of blood for a human as straight-walking creature. There is a background to examine it as physiological basis of forming of the hypertensive state [3, 4], including, for pregnant.

Figure 3 shows the subsequent dynamics of this setting for pregnancy in the first and second trimesters of PhP. It shows a clear reduction of the hypertensive states to their absence in the lying position, and it is especially shown in the upright position up to the third trimester. Such dynamics at PhP demonstrate optimization of the circulatory state of the CVS, at least on the mode of BPespecially it's important for maturing of pregnancy in terms of straight-walking (sitting, upright, at walking). Clear growth of expression of hypotonic states is thus marked in the lying position, with 10% for nonpregnant women (control group) to the first (39%) and the second trimesters - 32% ($P < 0.01$).

Figure 1 shows less expressed marked orientation in distribution of the modes for BP in the upright position determined at PaP. The hypertensive state is absent only in the first trimester. It appears in the second and third trimesters, though at lower levels (3–5%; $P \leq 0.05$) compared to nonpregnant women (10%). For PaP, the hypertensive states are present in the lying position during all three trimesters, increasing three times (from 5% for nonpregnant women to 15% in PaP; $P < 0.05$).

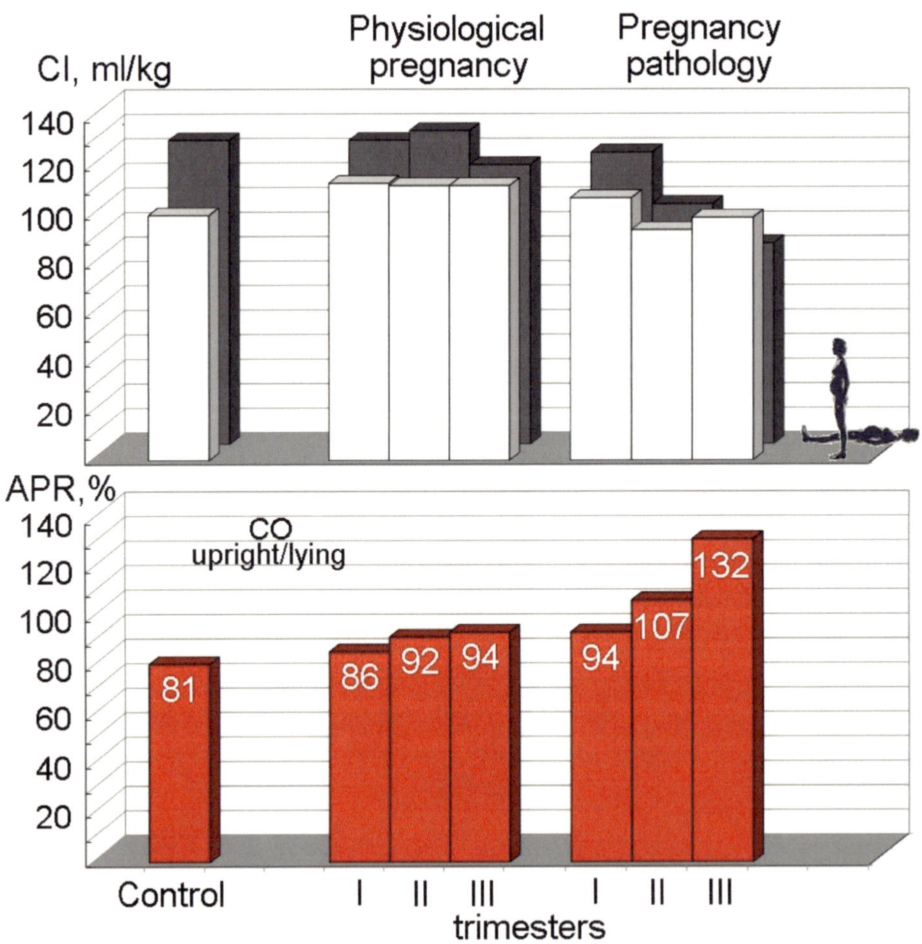

Figure 3.
Dynamics of the hemodynamic providing of physiological pregnancy (PhP) and pathological pregnancy (PP) on a cardiac index (CI = CO/kg body weight) in the lying and upright positions (marked by figures) and on antropophysiological correlation (APR = CO upright/lying, in %)—Index of typology alteration of dynamic organization of the CVS.

It should be noted, that according to optimization of the state of the CVS on the mode of BP for pregnant raising of systolic function of heart, especially clearly expressed at physiological pregnancy, was marked. **Table 1** presents the data on MBV, on positions lying SI and APF and upright in the first, second, and third trimesters of pregnancy. For analysis, we used an average ($X \pm m_x$) and non-parametric statistical descriptions of hemodynamic parameters: median (*Me*) and percentile range. The *k*-value of percentile was determined with 95% probability

Status	Bodyweight	CO, ml		APR, %	Cl, ml/kg	
		Lying	Standing		Lying	Standing
Nonpregnant women						
Women (of even-aged control group) n = 114	58	7164	5668	81	124	700
	51–56	5240–9255	4620–6974	64–100	88–157	79–123
	59 ± 1	7225 ± 222	5779 ± 186	84 ± 3	126 ± 3	100 ± 3
Physiological pregnancy (PhP)						
First trimester n = 23	65	8282	7018	86	124	113
	59–70	6204–15,581	6332–9323	70–123	78–181	73–144
	64 ± 1	9896 ± 585	7485 ± 211	91 ± 4	133 ± 9	116 ± 7
Increase of systolic descriptions—in 17 out of 20 ($P < 0.07$)						
Second trimester n = 38	62	7996	6788	92	128	112
	50–67	5837–11,130	5033–9408	79–109	77–175	81–150
	60 ± 1	7996 ± 344	6885 ± 229	94 ± 3	127 ± 6	114 ± 4
Increase of systolic descriptions—in 19 out of 20 ($P < 0.01$)						
Third trimester n = 53	71	9534	6640	94	114	103
	63–79	5264–10,528	5101–9536	86–103	77–146	78–145
	71 ± 1	7443 ± 242	7444 ± 225	112 ± 4	102 ± 4	108 ± 5
Increase of systolic descriptions—in 16 out of 20 ($P = 0.01$)						
Perinatal pathological with gestational endotheliopathy (PaP)						
First trimester n = 20	57	7754	7789	94	119	107
	49–62	5841–9297	4491–14,578	71–146	87–149	67–203
	56 ± 1	7840 ± 406	8809 ± 803	103 ± 8	125 ± 9	131 ± 14
Increase of systolic descriptions—in 14 out of 20 ($P = 0.05$)						
Second trimester n = 36	61	8019	7741	107	98	94
	56–69	5507–9428	6454–9817	84–135	64–157	65–160
	62 ± 1	7286 ± 419	7800 ± 480	106 ± 10	106 ± 9	110 ± 9
Increase of systolic descriptions—in 14 out of 20 ($P = 0.05$)						
Third trimester n = 75	68	5774	8305	132	82	99
	64–74	4075–6900	3615–9570	95–159	53–105	49–147
	69 ± 1	5730 ± 196	7128 ± 279	127 ± 5	84 ± 5	102 ± 4
Increase of systolic descriptions—in 9 out of 20 (*P*>)						

Statistical parameters of selection: the first row of digital data is a median (Me) of selection, second row is a percentile range (k_0–k_1) with 95% probability ($P \leq 0.05$), and the third row is an average by the c error of middle ($X \pm m_x$).

Table 1.
Cardiac output for nonpregnant women in control group and for pregnant women (first, second, and third trimesters).

($P \leq 0.05$) taking into account a sample size, percentile with $k \geq 0$ was determined as the lower limit of the percentile range, and $k \geq 1$ was determined as the higher limit. For convenience, shorthand signs will be used for -lower ($k0$) and overhead ($k1$) percentile.

MVB (minute volume of blood), APR (antropophysiological correlation), and CI (cardiac index) are homogeneous hemodynamic indexes and therefore they are taken for systole descriptions (parameters) of the hemodynamic providing of pregnancy on the pumping function of heart. A non-standard approach was used to estimate the differences of these descriptions in nonpregnant women (CG) and between PhP and PaP. Each one, of the estimated hemodynamic parameters (MBV, APF, and SI), as marked higher, on one or another condition (trimester, lying, upright) used, four descriptions, that is driven in **Figure 1** in order of their placement—*Me*, $k0$–$k1$, X.

Analyzing of the dynamics generally in all trimesters, was conducted by three hemodynamic criteria – MBV, CI (in a prone and standing position) and APR, in every separate trimester; a total number makes 20 descriptions. In comparison with a control group, and also PP and PaP, on non-parametric criteria; the amount of the descriptions is taken to the account with unidirectional difference (anymore, less than, absent).

Optimization of the circulatory state of the CVS during pregnancy accompanied by the clear increase of systolic descriptions on the pumping function of heart and shows up on all three trimesters, especially at PP (**Table 1**). On MBV such orientation simply shows up during all three trimesters as at PhP—lying and upright totally for 24 descriptions from 24 ($P < 0.01$) and at PaP—also for 18 from 24 ($P < 0.05$). However at development of pregnancy substantially, that the pumping function of heart provided increasing pregnant body and fetus weight, therefore the calculation of SI is oriented not to the surface of body of pregnant, but on its weight. Consideration of SI demonstrates clear weakness of systolic possibilities of the heart during PhP—in position lying on all 12 from 12 descriptions of SI lower as compared to nonpregnant, and for 11 from 12 descriptions lower as compared to PaP (see a **Table 1**). Unlike PhP at PaP the clear and increasing decline of SI was marked during all pregnancy (**Figure 3**), as compared to both nonpregnant women and PhP.

Unlike position of body lying—upright SI increases for 10 from 12 characteristics (totally for three trimesters) at PP ($P < 0.05$), while at PaP—only for 7 from 12 (P>). At this SI at PaP in position upright was for less comparing to PP—for 9 descriptions from 12 ($P < 0.05$). Should be noted clear change during pregnancy of correlation MBV upright/lying (in %) on the index of APF, which is the typological reflection of dynamic organization of the circulator state of CVS and demonstrated at pregnancy in position upright hyperkinetic alteration of pumping function of heart and circulatory state of the CVS. Thus, both on PhP and PaP—for 12 descriptions of APF from 12 ($P = 0.01$). However most expressed such alteration is in PaP, that totally during all three trimesters marked for 12 from 12 descriptions of APF ($P < 0.01$).

It should be noted that such alteration of typological structure of the circulator state of the CVS at pregnancy was marked at all general modes of BP (**Figure 2**). It's evident, that as compared to nonpregnant, stake of type III (in %) at PhP and PaP for increases at all three modes of BP ($P < 0.01$).

Thus at PaP it is greater comparing to PhP ($P < 0.01$), arriving at normotonic and hypertensive modes of BP of level of specific description on a selection—accordingly 66 and 76%. It is necessary to underline that both these modes of BP, unlike the hypotonic mode, are the reflection of pressor adjusting of the CVS. From the data presented on **Figure 4**, its evident, that at these modes of BP pressor orientation lowers representative hypokinetic state of the CVS (type I) with a decline MBV in position upright—to 10–12%.

It is necessary to mean that hemodynamic adaptation at pregnancy that was accompanied by increasing antigravity tension of CVS and that shows up in forming of the hyperkinetic state of MVB in position upright, from one side, directionally on the hemodynamic providing, increase of pumping function of heart; and, from another side, limits functional abilities of the CVS in type III.

In the conditions of such tension extreme depreciation of heart is real. Thus, there can be both the real clinical state developing during pregnancy (dystrophy, cardiomyopathy, ischemia, etc.) and hidden from standard diagnostic determination not clinically, and the hemodynamically identified transitory heart failure (tHF), as most early form of display of this state. Earlier we showed such possibility,

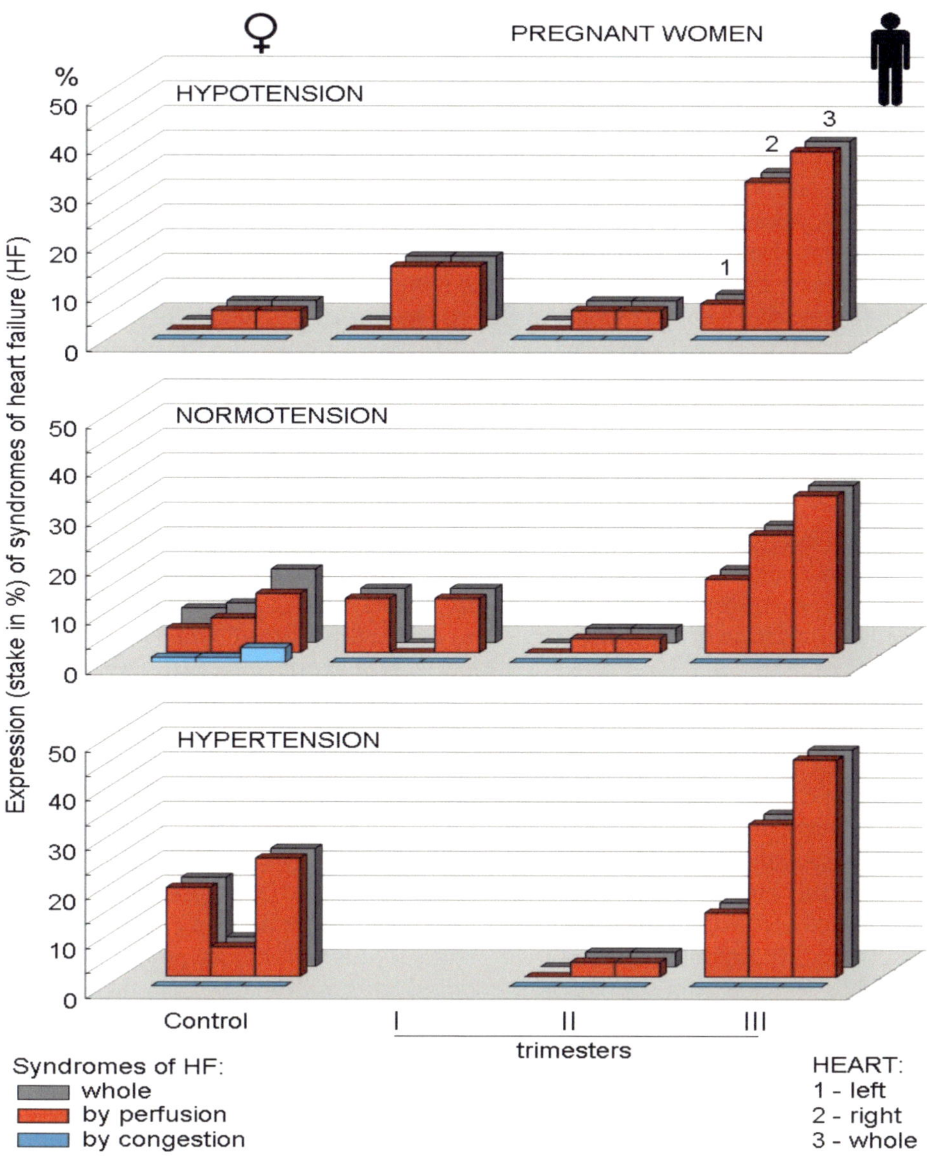

Figure 4.
Expression (stake in %) of syndromes of transitory heart failure (tHF) at the general modes of BP for women of reproductive age (control) and in the first, second, and third trimesters of pregnancy in the upright position.

including, in pregnancy [29], and also clear association of most expressive hemodynamic syndromes of insufficiency of circulation of blood is shown, including HF, exactly at type III of the circulatory state of CVS [30].

Thus it should be noted that at any modes of BP expression of hemodynamically identified HF for pregnant and nonpregnant women exactly in position upright—maximal antigravity tension of CVS, as compared to position lying, certainly higher (**Figure 5**).

So, if nonpregnant in control group in position lying in hypotonic, normotonic and hypertensive mode of expression of HF (stake in %) made about 0, 3 and 0%, then in position upright it increased in all three modes, accordingly to 4% ($P < 0.05$), 15% ($P < 0.01$) and 24% ($P < 0.05$). In general, but even more distinctly marked correlations on primary expression of tHF in position upright determined for pregnant. Thus, clearly growing from I to III trimester (**Figure 5**). It should be noted that all trimesters did not have any fundamental distinctions of expression of HF. An exception was made only by the hypertensive mode, which made expression of HF (50%) in II trimester, comparing to III trimester (44%).

Out of antigravity tension of CVS in lying position certain features showed up on different general modes of BP. So, at normotonic general orientation is traced—from the clear display of optimization of the circulatory state of CVS in I trimester with absence of CH to the increase of its expression in III trimester to 7% ($P = 0.05$). Absence of tHF in position lying for pregnant of "general" hypertensive mode and in II and in III trimesters attracts attention.

Another feature in position upright and lying of the circulatory state of CVS on the analyzable "general" modes of BP is differentiation of display of tHF on a right and left heart, and also on basic circulatory syndromes—on the syndrome of decline of arterial perfusion and syndrome of venous stagnation and insufficiency. From data presented in **Figure 4**, clearly evident, what for nonpregnant and pregnant (totally PhP and PaP) in position upright shows up mainly HF on a perfusion type, growing from the hypotonic mode to normotonic and, especially increasing at the hypertensive mode.

When it comes to pregnant, het real increase of expression of tHF in position upright in I trimester marked at the hypotonic state (**Figure 4**). On the whole dynamics on expression of HF in I and II trimesters of pregnancy reflects to the noted optimization of the circulatory state of CVS. Especially distinctly it shows up on II trimester, that is reflected in the low level of expression of HF. Substantial feature of the circulatory state of CVS at pregnancy in position upright is a primary display of right-heart tHF of perfusion type—on **Figure 4** practically on all positions, except pregnant with the normotonic mode. It's a sign that antigravity tension of CVS for pregnant in position upright the weakest links a right heart, consequently, pulmonary hemodynamics. As a result—growing pressure in the pulmonary artery and increased post-tension on the right ventricle.

Especially meaningful is the increase of expression of tHF in position upright determined in III trimester of pregnancy, including, and mainly on a right heart. Exactly on this stage of development of pregnancy the well-known physical terms, related to the increase of the sizes of uterus and fetus, maximally strengthen their synergistic influence on adjusting of circulation of blood on a gravitational (hydrostatical) factor and corresponding antigravity tension of CVS, directed of hemodynamic providing of pregnancy and actually organism of pregnant. It is necessary to remember, that dualism is real in this biologically important adaptation—not all, that is positive for the hemodynamic providing of fetoplacental complex, is positive for pregnant women. Actually, solving such dualism determines success of physiological development of pregnancy or pathological consequences during or afterwards.

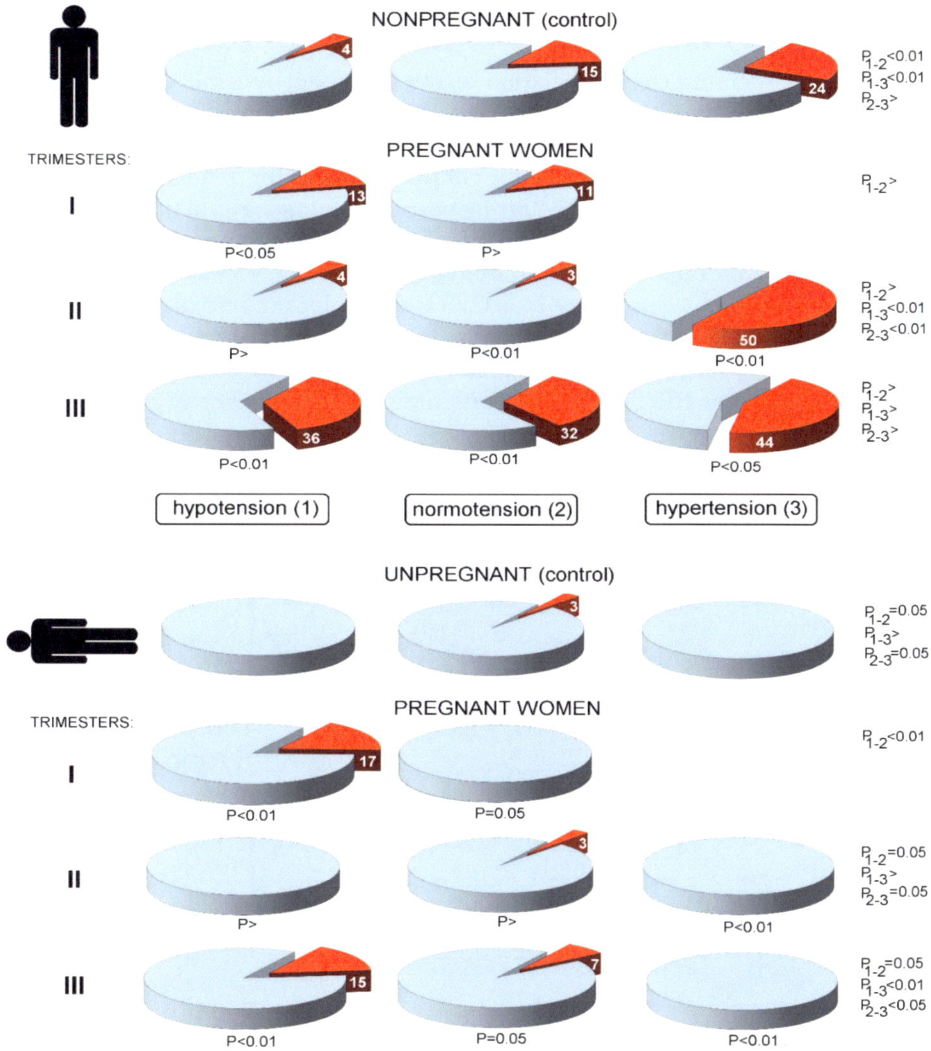

Figure 5.
General expression (stake in %) of syndromes of HF (total of left and right heart) for healthy nonpregnant women (control group) and on the general group of pregnant (total of PhP and PaP) at the "general" modes of the state of CVS for BP (hypotension, normotension, high blood pressure) in the upright and lying positions (marked by figures).

Practically one level of expression of tHF in III trimester at all examined general modes of BP testifies to independent meaning fullness to the PFH and syndrome of tHF in expression of antigravity tension of CVS and as possible circulatory basis of insufficiency of hemodynamic adaptation in pregnancy. It gives certain grounds to suppose that it's not in the mode of BP, and in structural organization of the circulatory state of CVS, functional basis of that is made by the pumping function of heart, and actually the state of last. Actually certain mode is the result of such alteration. Thus the marker of tension of hemodynamic alteration is a transition on the cardiac output to the hyperkinetic state in position upright comparing to lying—to type III of dynamic organization of the circulatory state of CVS, and by the predictor of insufficiency of adaptation of CVS, including, at pregnancy—results of hemodynamically identified by antropophysiological diagnostic algorithm of circulatory syndromes of HF. Last, as the most early circulator form of HF of perfusion type on preclinical level is a trigger of forming of dynamic organization of the circulatory state of CVS, corresponding to the hypertensive state, including, one in pregnancy.

Therefore, there is a clear association between tHF and dynamic alteration of the circulatory state of the CVS to the hyperkinetic condition (type III) in the upright position. On **Figure 6** at the same orientation of such alteration it is clearly determined higher stakes of type III, both for nonpregnant and for pregnant, exactly in a group with the syndromes of HF. During postnatal ontogenesis in the process of adaptation to the gravitational factor of circulation of blood, a transition to III to the type of dynamic organization of the circulator state of CVS was marked, that was accompanied by general growth on CVS and the blocks of circulation of blood of syndrome of the age-related depreciation (greater biological age) of the hemodynamically risky states, especially expressed at type III. Thus clearly grew expression of syndromes of HF. There are reasons to suppose that these two constituents

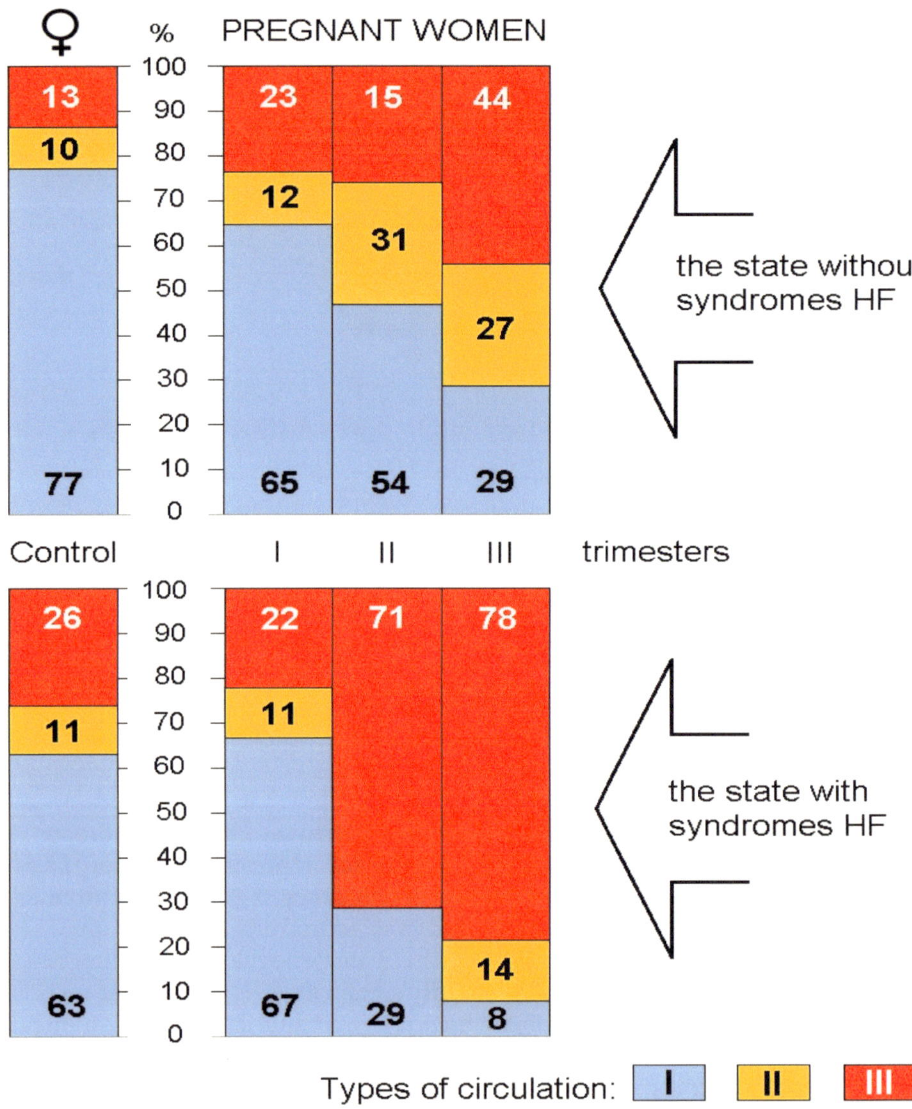

Figure 6.
Distribution of types of circulation (stake in % on a diagram) of blood on antropophysiological correlation of minute volume of blood (MVB) upright/lying—Hypokinetic (I), eukinetic (II), and hyperkinetic (III) in nonpregnant (control) women and pregnant women on the states with and without syndromes of tHF.

(typology alteration and HF) induce the features of dynamic organization of CVS at one or another somatic state.

Besides a trigger function, tHF was, as marked higher, by the display of antigravity tension of CVS, leading to functional depreciation of CVS and to increase of hemodynamic risk, both on the general state of circulation of blood and on the basic circulatory blocks of CVS.

At overlook of dynamic organization of the circulatory condition of CVS it is necessary to remember the state of the capacity making adjusting of CVS on the gravitational (hydrostatical) factor of circulation of blood, which is present in position upright, including for pregnant, in system vasoconstriction of arterial vessels, especially shown in vascular regions below level of heart [31]. It is necessary to notice, that in diagnostic algorithm as a syndrome of resistance, the state when indexes of arterial impedance (vascular resistance) exceed a normative increase, is fixed. Mentioned on **Figure 7** data clearly demonstrate the value of the state of heart in this system adjusting to pressor orientation, especially in position upright. Both for nonpregnant and pregnant those who have hemodynamically identified tHF, as a rule, perfusion type, in position upright marked more expressed (red blocks), as compared to the states without tHF (green blocks), system vasoconstriction. By grey color marked blocks of circulation of blood, on which distinctions are absent.

Optimization of the circulatory state of CVS during pregnancy by the regime of blood pressure, especially with FP, was accompanied by a clear overall increase in systolic characteristics of the PhP. This orientation in the cardiac minute volume (CMV, ml) unambiguously manifested itself during all three trimesters as with PhP—lying and standing in total according to 24 characteristics out of 24 ($P < 0.01$), while with gestational endotheliopathy—by 18 out of 24 ($P < 0.05$). If the manifestation of type III under hypotonic, normotonic, and hypertonic regimes in blood pressure was 8, 12, and 6%, respectively, then in case of PhP it was 21, 36, and 50%, respectively (for all P positions <0.01) and for PaP, 48, 66, and 76% (for all positions $P < 0.01$). For gestational endotheliopathy in all modes of blood pressure, the representativeness of the hyperkinetic state in the e pumping function of

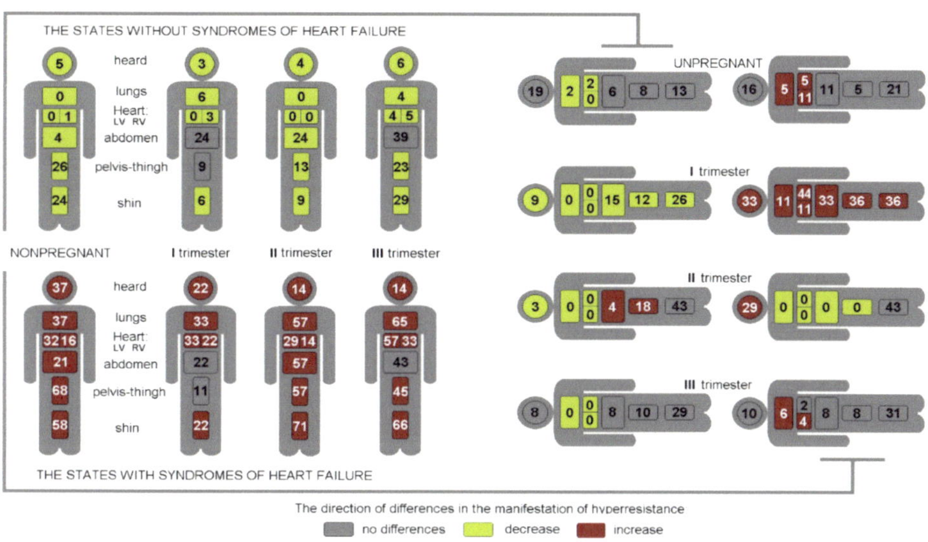

Figure 7.
Antropophysiological (upright and lying positions) characteristics of differences of expression (stake in %) of syndromes of hyperresistance of arterial vessels for nonpregnant (control) women and pregnant women at comparison on groups with syndromes of HF and without.

the heart standing (type III) was significantly higher compared to PhP ($P < 0.01$). According to it, the marker of tension of hemodynamic alteration was a transition on the CMV to the hyperkinetic state in position from standing to lying—to type III of dynamic organization of the circulator state of CVS and system hyperresistance of arterial vessels, and by the predictor of insufficiency of adaptation of CVS was displayed mostly in the position upright by perfusion type, combining with circulatory syndromes limiting adaptive possibilities of arterial circulation.

For hemodynamic providing of pregnancy such system of vasoconstriction has a critical value, especially for circulatory blocks, directly responsible for hemodynamic providing of fetoplacental link—abdominal and pelvic circulation of blood. Placenta, volume of amniotic fluid, and self-weight of fetus in max decrease influence of gravitational (hydrostatical) pressure at straight-walking (sitting, upright, walking). However direct dependence of the hemodynamic providing of fetoplacental complex from maternal circulation of blood is saved, both from regional, especially abdominal and pelvic and the circulatory state of CVS in general and its central link—pumping function of heart [32].

Expression of autonomic "slipping out" of arterial vessels of abdominal and pelvic circulation from under system vasoconstriction, probably because of endothelium-depending humoral mechanism, determine phenomenon of optimization of the circulatory state of CVS at the beginning of pregnancy, especially expressed at PhP, and inhibition of pathological changes. And, vice versa, expressed vasoconstriction of abdominal and pelvic arterial vessels, along with hypoperfusion and decrease of pumping function of heart determine circulatory basis of PaP (in the first place preeclampsia). Therefore, estimating the circulatory state of CVS for pregnant, and nonpregnant, necessary to be oriented not on the mode of BP, but on condition of basic perfusion mechanisms a "volume of blood—pumping function of heart—vascular capacity—blood stream" and regulators of autonomic regional blood flow—endothelial function providing distribution of peripheral circulation of blood, and it explained that gestational endotheliopathy is the trigger component of disorder hemodynamics supply pregnancy and development of perinatal pathology. In fact, the state of perfusion mechanisms that form the basis of hemodynamic support of any somatic condition and especially pregnancy, taking into account the formation of a fetoplacental complex «above organism» and necessity of hemodynamic adaptation of CVS of pregnant as straight-walking creature, to formed exceptional organism situation not only in gestational feature, but also in aspect of adaptation.

4. Conclusions

1. The typological transition in the dynamic organization of the circulatory state of the CVS by CO to the hyperkinetic state in the standing relative to the lying position (type III) and the manifestation of systemic hyperresistance of arterial vessels reflects the tension of adaptation of the CVS during hemodynamic support of pregnancy.

2. The predictor of insufficiency of adaptation of the CVS during hemodynamic support of pregnancy, especially with PaP, is gestational endotheliopathy. Playing a role of a trigger, for manifestation of a hemodynamic syndrome of HF in a perfusion type, which is predominantly in a standing position, combined with circulatory syndromes that limit the adaptive capabilities of arterial circulation (hyperresistance, ischemia), which is especially relevant for abdominal and pelvic circulation.

3. Hemodynamically identified HF by perfusion type, as the earliest circulatory form at the preclinical level for gestational endotheliopathy, is considered a trigger for the formation of a dynamic organization of the circulatory state of the CVS corresponding to the hypertensive state, including during pregnancy (preeclampsia).

Funding

The authors received no financial support for the research, authorship, and/or publication of this article.

Conflict of interest

The authors declare no conflict of interest.

Author details

Dmytro Konkov[1], George Belkania[2], Levon Dilenyan[3], Victor Rud[1], Liana Puchalska[4], Alina Piskun[1] and Larisa Klimas[1]*

1 National Pirogov Memorial Medical University, Vinnytsya, Ukraine

2 Expert Medical System Laboratory, Vinnytsya, Ukraine

3 Privolzhsky Research Medical University, Nizhny Novgorod, Russia

4 University of Warsaw, Department of Experimental and Clinical Physiology Warsaw, Poland

*Address all correspondence to: lora@vnmu.edu.ua

References

[1] Ridder A, Giorgione V, Khalil A, Thilaganathan B. Preeclampsia: The relationship between uterine artery blood flow and trophoblast function. International Journal of Molecular Sciences. 2019;**20**(13):3263. DOI: 10.3390/ijms20133263

[2] Thilaganathan B. Pre-eclampsia and the cardiovascular–placental axis. Ultrasound in Obstetrics & Gynecology. 2018;**51**(6):714-717. DOI: 10.1002/uog.19081

[3] Konkov DG, Belkania GS, Puchalska LG. The modern hemodynamic features of predictive diagnosis of preeclampsia. In: The Abstract Book of the 18th World Congress of the Gynecological Endocrinology; 7-10 March 2018; Florence, Italy; 2018. p. 214

[4] Borzenko I, Konkov D, Kondratova I, Basilayshvili O, Gargin V. Influence of endotheliopathy of spiral arteries on placental ischemia. Georgian Medical News. 2019;**11**(296):131-134

[5] Konkov DG, Piskun AO. The features of placental angiogenesis in early preeclampsia. Actual Questions of Modern Gynecology and Perinatology. 2018;**5**(4):25-29

[6] Konkov DG. The features of conversion of spiral arteries in pregnant women with the gestational endotheliopathy. Reports of Vinnytsia National Medical University. 2016; **20**(1):65-68

[7] Kalafat E, Thilaganathan B. Cardiovascular origins of preeclampsia. Current Opinion in Obstetrics and Gynecology. 2017;**29**(6):383-389. DOI: 10.1097/GCO.0000000000000419

[8] Coutinho T, Lamai O, Nerenberg K. Hypertensive disorders of pregnancy and cardiovascular diseases: Current knowledge and future directions. Current Treatment Options in Cardiovascular Medicine. 2018;**20**(7):56. DOI: 10.1007/s11936-018-0653-8

[9] Thilaganathan B, Kalafat E. Cardiovascular system in preeclampsia and beyond. Hypertension. 2019;**73**(3):522-531. DOI: 10.1161/HYPERTENSIONAHA.118.11191

[10] Konkov DG. The features of circulatory dynamics during physiological pregnancy. Reports of Morphology. 2012;**18**(2):317-321

[11] Konkov DG, Belkaniya GS, Dilenyan LR, et al. The multidisciplinary point of view on the condition of hemodynamic maintenance of pregnancy the anthropophysiological approach. Ohrana materinstva i detstva. 2017;**1**(29):5-13

[12] Belkaniya G, Konkov D, Dilenyan L, et al. The anthropophysiologic characteristics of circulatory model of haemodynamic pregnancy supporting. Reproductive Health. Eastern Europe. 2018;**8**(1):55-75

[13] Belkaniya GS, Dilenyan LR, Bagrii AS, et al. General approaches to anthropophysiologica of characterization of age-related changes in human circulation. Patogenez. 2017;**15**(4):24-31

[14] Belkaniya GS, Konkov DG, Dilenyan LR, et al. The anthropophysiological analisis of systemic vasoconstruction and endothelio-dependent vasodilation in the hemodynamic supplying of pregnancy. Actual Questions of Modern Gynecology and Perinatology. 2018;**5**(1):30-41

[15] Belkaniia GS. Funktsional'naia sistema antigravitatsii [Functional antigravitation system]. Problemy Kosmicheskoĭ Biologii. 1982;**45**:5-286

[16] Belkaniia GS, Dartsmeliia VA. Priamokhozhdenie kak faktor razvitiia arterial'noĭ gipertonii u primatov [Upright walking as a factor in the development of arterial hypertension in primates]. Kosmicheskaia Biologiia i Aviakosmicheskaia Meditsina. 1984;**18**(3):14-19

[17] Belkaniya GS, Dilenyan LR, Bagriy AS, et al. Kardiodinamicheskie osnovyi i perspektivyi klinicheskogo ispolzovaniya reografii [The cardiodynamic basis and prospects for clinical use of rheography. Anthropophysiological aspect]. Nizhniy Novgorod: izd-vo Nizhegorodskoy gosudarstvennoy meditsinskoy akademi; 2016. p. 220

[18] Belkaniya GS, Dilenyan LR, Bagriy AS, et al. Antropofiziologicheskiy podhod v formirovanii diagnosticheskoy shkalyi gemodinamicheskih parametrov [The anthropophysiological approach in the formation of a diagnostic scale of hemodynamic parameters]. Meditsinskiy almanah. 2014;**2**(32): 152-156

[19] Dartsmeliia VA, Belkaniia GS. Tipologicheskaia kharakteristika gemodinamicheskikh sostoianiĭ v ortostatike u zdorovykh lits [Typological characteristics of hemodynamic states in the orthostatism of healthy persons]. Kosmicheskaia Biologiia i Aviakosmicheskaia Meditsina. 1985;**19**(2):26-33

[20] Dilenyan LR, Belkaniya GS, Bagriy AS, et al. Antropofiziologicheskiy podhod v sistemnom algoritme kriterialnogo analiza sostoyaniya serdechno-sosudistoy sistemyi [The anthropophysiological approach in the system algorithm of criteria analysis of the state of the cardiovascular system]. Meditsinskiy almanah. 2014;**5**(35): 170-174

[21] Dilenyan LR, Belkaniya GS, Bagriy AS, et al. Sindromalnyiy analiz krovoobrascheniya v sistemnom algoritme antropofiziologicheskogo isssledovaniya [The syndromic analysis of the state of the cardiovascular system]. Meditsinskiy almanah. 2015;**1**(36):125-130

[22] Belkaniya GS, Dilenyan LR, Ryzhakov DI, et al. Diagnostic informativity of hemodynamic identification of circulatory syndromes in heart failure. Patogenez. 2017; **15**(3):84-92

[23] Belkaniya GS, Dilenyan LR, Bagriy AS, et al. Osobennosti metodicheskogo obespecheniya antropofiziologicheskoy diagnostiki sostoyaniya serdechno-sosudistoysistemyi [The features of methodological support anthropophysiological diagnostics of the condition of cardio-vascular system]. Meditsinskiy almanah. 2013;**6**(30):208-214

[24] Dilenyan LR, Bagriy AS, Belkaniya GS, et al. Antro pogeneticheskaya model vozrastnoy dinamiki regulyatornoy ustanovki tsirkulyatornogo sostoyaniya serdechno-sosudistoy sistemyi [Anthropophysiological characteristics of«hemodynamic model»of age dynamics of circulation in humans]. Sovremennyie problemyi nauki i obrazovaniya. 2015;**6**:1-30

[25] Dilenyan LR, Belkaniya GS, Bagriy AS, et al. Antropofiziologi cheskaya harakteristika tipologicheskogo otrazheniya obschey sindromalnoy strukturyi tsirkulyatornogo sostoyaniya serdechno-sosudistoy sistemyi [Anthropophysiological characteristics of typological reflection of general structure of the cardiovascular system]. Sovremennyie problemyi nauki i obrazovaniya. 2016;**3**:1-34

[26] Belkaniya GS, Konkov DG, Dilenyan LR, et al. Novyiy vzglyad na

krovoobraschenie u beremennyih—antropofiziologicheskaya diagnostika gemodinamicheskogo obespecheniya beremennosti [A new look at the circulation in pregnant women—anthropophysiligical diagnostics of hemodynamic support of pregnancy]. Sovremennyie problemyi nauki i obrazovaniya. 2017;**5**:1-18

[27] Belkaniya GS, Dartsmeliya VA, Galustyan MV, et al. Anthro pophysiological basis of species-specific stereotype of cardiovascular system reactivity in primates. Vestnik AMN SSSR. 1987;**10**:52-60

[28] Genes VS. Nekotoryie prostyie metodyi kiberneticheskoy obrabotki dannyih diagnosticheskih i fiziologicheskih issledovaniy [Some simple methods of cybernetic processing of diagnostic and physiological research data]. M.: Nauka; 1967. p. 208

[29] Belkaniya GS, Dilenyan LR, Konkov DG, et al. An anthropogenic model of cardiovascular system adaptation to the Earth's gravity as the conceptual basis of pathological anthropology. Journal of Physiological Anthropology. 2021;**40**(1):9. DOI: 10.1186/s40101-021-00260-2

[30] Dilenyan LR, Belkaniya GS, Martusevich AK. Role of systemic vasoconstruction in regulatory installation of blood circulation. Journal of Stress Physiology Biochemistry. 2018;**14**(4):35-45

[31] Belkaniia GS. Funktsional'naia sistema antigravitatsii i modelirovanie fiziologicheskikh éffektov ponizhennoĭ gravitatsii [Functional antigravitational system and modeling the physiological effects of reduced gravity]. Uspekhi Fiziologicheskikh Nauk. 1978; **9**(2):103-128

[32] Belkaniya GS, Dilenyan LR, Bagriy AS, et al. Antropofiziologi cheskoe obosnovanie tipologicheskogo opredeleniya optimalnosti i neoptimalnosti gemodinamicheskogo obespecheniya somaticheskogo sostoyaniya organizma [The anthropophysiological substantiation of the typological definition of the hemodynamic supply of the organism]. Meditsinskiy almanah. 2014;**1**(31): 119-122

Section 6

Opthalamic Disorder

Chapter 6

Ophthalmic Disorders in Posterior Reversible Encephalopathy Syndrome Associated with Preeclampsia

Katarina Cvitkovic, Anita Pusic Sesar, Antonio Sesar and Ivan Cavar

Abstract

Posterior reversible encephalopathy syndrome (PRES) is a clinicoradiological entity presented with different symptoms such as visual disturbances, headaches, seizures, severe hypertension and altered mental status. It has been recognized in a different pathological conditions, although preeclampsia/eclampsia is the most common cause of PRES. The pathogenesis of PRES is still not fully understood, but it seems that failure of cerebrovascular autoregulation causing vasogenic edema, cerebral vasoconstriction, and disruption of the blood brain barrier plays an important role. Cortical blindness, hypertensive retinopathy, serous retinal detachment (SRD), central retinal artery and vein occlusions, retinal or vitreous hemorrhages, anterior ischemic optic neuropathy (AION) and Purtscher's retinopathy are ophthalmic disorders that may occur in PRES associated with preeclampsia. Among these, cortical blindness is the best documented complication of preeclampsia. Magnet resonance imaging (MRI) is a gold standard to establish the diagnosis of PRES because clinical findings are not sufficiently specific. Typically, there are bilateral cortical occipital lesions with hyperdensity on T2-weighted MRI. Blindness due to occipital lesions is reversible and the vision loss is usually regained within 4 h to 8 days.

Keywords: preeclampsia, eclampsia, posterior reversible encephalopathy syndrome, ophthalmological disorders, cortical blindness

1. Introduction

Posterior reversible encephalopathy syndrome (PRES) is a clinicoradiological entity presented with different symptoms, such as headaches, seizures, visual disturbances, severe hypertension, and altered mental status [1]. Previously, it has been known by various names such as reversible posterior leukoencephalopathy syndrome, reversible posterior cerebral edema syndrome, and reversible occipital parietal encephalopathy [2, 3]. PRES was first described in 1996 by Hinchey et al. in patients with acute neurological symptoms and since then it has been recognized in different pathological conditions such as preeclampsia, eclampsia, hypertensive encephalopathy, autoimmune diseases, renal failure, infection, and the use of cytotoxic or immunosuppressive drugs [1, 3–9]. Among these, preeclampsia and eclampsia are the most common causes of PRES. Preeclampsia is pregnancy-specific disorder clinically characterized by a new onset of hypertension and proteinuria that appear after the 20th week of gestation and up to 6 weeks postpartum in a previously normotensive woman [5, 6]. Preeclampsia and its variants affect approximately 5% of pregnancies and is the leading cause of both maternal and fetal morbidity and mortality worldwide [10]. It is characterized by impaired organ perfusion that occurs as a result of vasospasm and activation of the coagulation system [11]. Eclampsia is an acute cerebral complication of preeclampsia, presented with the occurrence of tonic-clonic convulsions in pregnant or recently postpartum women [12]. Severe intracranial vasospasm, local ischemia, intracranial hypertension, and endothelial dysfunction associated with vasogenic and cytotoxic edema are possible causes of seizures in PRES [11]. Rare cases of PRES in pregnant women with normal blood pressure and without preeclampsia have also been described in the literature [13]. Early recognition of PRES is essential in order to timely apply the medication, which typically includes drugs that lower blood pressure, act as anti-edematous and interrupt tonic-clonic convulsions [7].

2. Pathogenesis of PRES

The exact pathophysiological mechanisms of PRES are not precisely known. Failure of cerebrovascular autoregulation, cerebral vasoconstriction, and disruption of the blood brain barrier due to endothelial disfunction are possible mechanisms involved in the pathogenesis of PRES [2]. Failure of cerebrovascular autoregulation causing vasogenic edema is the most accepted one. It seems that hyperperfusion plays a crucial role in disorders where hypertension is a key feature, such as in preeclampsia [14]. During fluctuations of systemic blood pressure, cerebrovascular autoregulation maintains cerebral blood flow, leading to vasodilation during systemic hypotension and vasoconstriction during systemic hypertension. The rapid development of hypertension can exceed the capacity of cerebral blood flow autoregulation leading to hyperperfusion [14]. It is supposed that posterior brain regions are more vulnerable to hyperperfusion, which is explained by better autoregulation of the anterior circulation due to better sympathetic innervations as compared to the posterior circulation [15]. Another theory suggests spasm of cerebral arteries in response to acute hypertension, thus resulting in decreased cerebral blood flow, intraarterial thrombosis, and cerebral ischemia leading to cytotoxic edema, especially in the border zones between arterial territories [16–18]. Breakdown of the blood brain barrier and endothelial dysfunction occurs in PRES with fluid and macromolecule extravasation into the interstitium. Further, increased concentrations of circulating cytokines activate endothelial cells and allow adhesion of circulating leukocytes. On the other hand, the tight junctions are disrupted and vascular endothelial growth factor expression is increased, leading to increased vascular permeability and vasogenic edema [19].

3. Neuroimaging features of PRES

The diagnosis of PRES cannot be established exclusively on clinical findings [1]. Brain lesions are usually located in the white matter, although rarely, overlying cortex may also be affected [20]. The parieto-occipital regions of the brain are main foci of changes, that are usually bilateral and symmetric. However, the lesions can also extend to other brain structures such as the frontal and temporal lobes, cerebellar hemispheres, basal ganglia, brain stem, and deep white matter [21]. A multislice computed tomography (MSCT) scan is often normal or shows cortical-subcortical hypodensities, predominantly in posterior brain regions. However, MSCT scans in PRES show lesions in only of about 50% cases [22]. Because of that, magnet resonance imaging (MRI) is a gold standard for the diagnosis of PRES and the follow-up of these patients. Neuroimaging studies showed hypointense or isointense signal changes on T1-weighted images. The typical neuroimaging feature is a high signal intensity on T2-weighted images predominantly in the posterior regions, which is caused by subcortical white matter vasogenic edema [1]. Abnormalities are more observable on fluid-attenuated inversion recovery imaging (FLAIR), which increases the ability to detect subtle lesions in PRES [15]. Supplemental diffusion-weighted imaging (DWI) and apparent diffusion coefficient (ADC) map images are helpful in distinguishing vasogenic oedema from cytotoxic edema [15–19]. Cytotoxic edema appears hyperintense on DWI with a low signal intensity image on the corresponding ADC sequence. A predominantly low signal on DWI and a high signal on ADC image indicates vasogenic edema. Vasogenic edema and cytotoxic edema can also coexist in eclampsia [23].

4. Ocular disorders in PRES associated with preeclampsia

Visual disorders in pregnancy can be highly variable and range from mild symptoms such as transient blurred vision, photopsia, and different types of visual field defects to transient or permanent total blindness [24]. Vision loss during pregnancy has been documented in 1–3% of cases and a possible causes are cortical blindness, central retinal artery and vein occlusions, retinal detachment, ischemic optic neuropathy, retinal or vitreous hemorrhages, and Purtscher's retinopathy [24–26]. Approximately 25% patients with severe preeclampsia and 50% patients with eclampsia present different visual symptoms including blurred vision, homonymous hemianopsia, visual neglect, visual anosognosia, and cortical blindness [27, 28]. They seem to be a consequence of the cerebral edema located in the occipital cortex or in the temporal and parietal association cortices. In most patients, the visual impairment is reversible, but in rare cases, permanent blindness has been described [29].

4.1 Cortical blindness

Cortical blindness is among the best-documented complications of preeclampsia/eclampsia and affects almost 15% of eclamptic women [30, 31]. Cortical blindness is caused by a dysfunction in the visual pathway that conducts visual information from the lateral geniculate nucleus of the thalamus to the cerebral visual cortex [20]. Vasogenic edema is the main cause of cortical blindness. It appears that the primary visual cortex in the occipital lobes is more susceptible to the breakdown of cerebrovascular autoregulation and subsequent hyperperfusion than other brain regions [31]. Cortical blindness has been described to occur several hours before or after eclamptic seizures, rarely several days or weeks postpartum [32–34]. The bilateral vision loss often begins with blurry vision and progresses within a couple of hours to bare light perception [35]. Sometimes, the woman is unaware of her blindness and feels that she can see, which is known as visual anosognosia or Anton syndrome, indicating involvement of the visual association cortex [34, 36]. However, cortical blindness is associated with an intact pathway from the eye to the lateral geniculate body and therefore ophthalmological examination including the pupillary reflexes, ocular motility, and fundoscopic findings is normal in these patients [29]. Blindness due to occipital lesions is reversible and the vision loss is usually regained within 4 h to 8 days [27].

5. Other ocular disorders in pregnancy complicated with preeclampsia

5.1 Hypertensive retinopathy

According to some studies, the prevalence rate of hypertensive retinopathy in women with hypertensive disorders in pregnancy is 32.5% [37]. Generally, the retinal vascular changes correlate with the severity of systemic hypertension. At the pathophysiological level, increased blood pressure leads to focal or diffuse vasoconstriction. In addition, increased vascular permeability leads to the extravasation of fluid to the extravascular spaces. Clinically, the most common abnormality seen during fundoscopy is narrowing of retinal arterioles [38]. Other retinal changes that may be present are decreased retinal artery to vein ratio, cotton wool spots, hemorrhages and Elschnig spots [39]. Vasospastic manifestations are reversible, and the retinal vessels rapidly return to normal after delivery [38].

5.2 Serous retinal detachment

Serous retinal detachment (SRD) is a rare complication of hypertensive disease in pregnancy, affecting 1–2% of preeclamptic and 10% of eclamptic women [40]. It is characterized by separation of the neurosensory retina from the pigmented retinal epithelium and it is usually observed in the absence of significant retinal vascular abnormalities or retinal breaks [41]. It may be present either before or after delivery [42]. Clinically, patients report loss of visual acuity and visual field defects [42, 43]. The detachments are often bullous and bilateral [27]. The exact pathophysiology of SRD in cases of preeclampsia is not well known, but it seems to be related with choroidal ischemia, which is secondary to an intensive arteriolar vasospasm [27]. The choroidal vascular insufficiency can lead to lesions in retinal pigment epithelium, fluid transudation, and focal retinal detachment. The majority of women who manifest SRD during pregnancy have a gradually improvement of visual acuity in few weeks after delivery, ending with complete recovery of vision [31]. Management of SRD in preeclampsia is conservative and involves treating the underlying condition [27].

5.3 Purtscher's retinopathy

Purtscher's retinopathy is a rare cause of visual loss during pregnancy and has been mostly described in association with complicated labor [24]. However, isolated cases during normal spontaneous labor have also been described in the literature [44]. Clinically, it presents with decreased visual acuity and a different types of visual field defects such as central or paracentral scotoma. The retinal changes include ischemia at the posterior pole with white patches of edema known as Purtscher's flecken, which represent areas of capillary bed infarction. In the initial phase, the optic disc is normal, but in the later phases, disc pallor and optic atrophy occur [27]. According to some researchers, these fundoscopic changes may be caused by embolic occlusion of the precapillary arterioles of the retina by fat, air, platelets, and leukocyte aggregates [45, 46]. The diagnosis is established on the basis of clinical findings and confirmed by intravenous fluorescein angiography [47]. The majority of patients recover some of their visual function without treatment. Use of systemic steroids may improve visual outcome in some patients, but momentary specific medication is not available [47].

5.4 Anterior ischemic optic neuropathy

Anterior ischemic optic neuropathy (AION) is a rare ophthalmological disorder in preeclampsia that has been described to occur before and after delivery. Clinically, it is presented with sudden vision loss and unilateral or bilateral disc edema [48, 49]. The exact pathophysiology of AION in preeclampsia remains unclear, but it is suggested that uncontrolled hypertension leads to vasoconstriction or ischemia in the posterior ciliary artery circulation [49].

5.5 Central retinal vein occlusion

Central retinal vein occlusion (CRVO) is also described in preeclamptic women and was presented with bilateral vision loss up to 21 days postpartum. Ophthalmologic examination reveals multiple retinal hemorrhages in all 4 quadrants, venous dilatation, and macular edema. Improvement of visual acuity is significant but not complete [31]. The exact pathophysiological mechanism of CRVO in preeclampsia is not fully understood; however, it is proposed that central retinal artery thickening is thought to cause compression of the central retinal vein, thereby leading to venous occlusion [50, 51].

5.6 Central retinal artery occlusion

Central retinal artery occlusion (CRAO) is rare in young people, and it is usually associated with a predisposing pathological disorders such as cardiac valvular disease, systemic vascular disease, and hypercoagulable disorders. According to some studies, CRAO is rarely described in women with eclampsia [52, 53]. Clinically, it is presented with sudden, painless, and persistent vision loss. Fundoscopy shows typical changes such as pallor of posterior pole with cherry-red spot. It seems that the activation of coagulation system could be a cause of multiple emboli and vascular occlusion in these patients [53].

5.7 Retinal and vitreous hemorrhages

Retinal and vitreous hemorrhages are rare disorders that may precede the appearance of preeclampsia. They are presented as a sudden vision loss in a normotensive pregnant women, who usually develop preeclampsia within 2 weeks after labor [54, 55].

6. Conclusion

Preeclampsia and eclampsia are the most common conditions associated with PRES. Due to the high predilection of pathological lesions in white matter of the occipital lobes, PRES could be manifested with different types of ocular disorders. Some of these complications can be serious including cortical blindness, SRD, CRVO, CRAO, AION, and vitreal and retinal hemorrhages. Clinicians should be aware of these ocular manifestations, and careful ophthalmological, neurological, and neuroradiological evaluation should be carried out to ascertain the various causes of vision loss in pregnancy. In most cases, visual prognosis is usually good with permanent vision recovery. Effective treatment of preeclampsia/eclampsia along with termination of pregnancy is the mainstay of treatment.

Conflict of interest

The authors declare they do not have any conflict of interest.

Author details

Katarina Cvitkovic[1,2]*, Anita Pusic Sesar[2], Antonio Sesar[2] and Ivan Cavar[1,2]

1 Department of Immunology, School of Medicine, University of Mostar, Mostar, Bosnia and Herzegovina

2 Department of Ophthalmology, University Hospital Center, Mostar, Bosnia and Herzegovina

*Address all correspondence to: katarina.cvitkovic@mef.sum.ba

References

[1] Lamy C, Oppenheim C, Méder JF, Mas JL. Neuroimaging in posterior reversible encephalopathy syndrome. Journal of Neuroimaging. 2004;**14**:89-96

[2] Sudulagunta SR, Sodalagunta MB, Kumbhat M, Settikere NA. Posterior reversible encephalopathy syndrome (PRES). Oxford Medical Case Reports. 2017;**2017**:omx011. DOI: 10.1093/omcr/omx011

[3] Bartynski WS. Posterior reversible encephalopathy syndrome, part 1: Fundamental imaging and clinical features. AJNR. American Journal of Neuroradiology. 2008;**29**:1036-1042. DOI: 10.3174/ajnr.A0928

[4] Hinchey J, Chaves C, Appignani B, Breen J, Pao L, Wang A, et al. A reversible posterior leukoencephalopathy syndrome. The New England Journal of Medicine. 1996;**334**:494-500. DOI: 10.1056/NEJM199602223340803

[5] Staykov D, Schwab S. Posterior reversible encephalopathy syndrome. Der Nervenarzt. 2012;**83**:1013-1020. DOI: 10.1007/s00115-012-3480-2

[6] Zeeman GG. Neurologic complications of pre-eclampsia. Seminars in Perinatology. 2009;**33**:166-172. DOI: 10.1053/j.semperi.2009.02.003

[7] Postma IR, Slager S, Kremer HP, de Groot JC, Zeeman GG. Long-term consequences of the posterior reversible encephalopathy syndrome in eclampsia and preeclampsia: A review of the obstetric and nonobstetric literature. Obstetrical & Gynecological Survey. 2014;**69**:287-300. DOI: 10.1097/OGX.0000000000000069

[8] Nielsen LH, Grén BS, Ovesen PG. Posterior reversible encephalopathy syndrome postpartum. Clinical Case Reports. 2015;**3**:266-270. DOI: 10.1002/ccr3.218

[9] Richards CR, McMurray RC, Criman ET, Clark ME, Gillern S. An unusual presentation of a rare disease: Posterior reversible encephalopathy syndrome following abdominal sepsis. Journal of Surgical Case Reports. 2016;**2016**:rjw184. DOI: 10.1093/jscr/rjw184

[10] Wagner SJ, Acquah LA, Lindell EP, Craici IM, Wingo MT, Rose CH, et al. Posterior reversible encephalopathy syndrome and eclampsia: Pressing the case for more aggressive blood pressure control. Mayo Clinic Proceedings. 2011;**86**:851-856. DOI: 10.4065/mcp.2011.0090

[11] Neligan PJ, Laffey JG. Clinical review: Special populations—Critical illness and pregnancy. Critical Care. 2011;**15**:227. DOI: 10.1186/cc10256

[12] Bo QY, Zhao XH, Yang X, Wang SJ. Reversible posterior encephalopathy syndrome associated with late onset postpartum eclampsia: A case report. Experimental and Therapeutic Medicine. 2016;**12**:1885-1888. DOI: 10.3892/etm.2016.3533

[13] Fujiwara Y, Higaki H, Yamada T, Nakata Y, Kato S, Yamamoto H, et al. Two cases of reversible posterior leukoencephalopathy syndrome, one with and the other without pre-eclampsia. The Journal of Obstetrics and Gynaecology Research. 2005;**31**:520-526. DOI: 10.1111/j.1447-0756.2005.00345.x

[14] Gewirtz AN, Gao V, Parauda SC, Robins MS. Posterior reversible encephalopathy yyndrome. Current Pain and Headache Reports. 2021;**25**:19. DOI: 10.1007/s11916-020-00932-1

[15] Schwartz RB, Feske SK, Polak JF, et al. Preeclampsia-eclampsia: Clinical and neuroradiographic correlates and insight into the pathogenesis of hypertensive encephalopathy.

Radiology. 2000;**217**:371-376. DOI: 10.1148/radiology.217.2.r00nv44371

[16] Henderson RD, Rajah T, Nicol AJ, Read SJ. Posterior leukoencephalopathy following intrathecal chemotherapy with MRA-documented vasospam. Neurology. 2003;**60**:326-328. DOI: 10.1212/01.wnl.0000042095.49520.1e

[17] Schwartz RB, Mulkern RV, Gudbjartsson H, Jolesz F. Diffusion-weighted MR imaging in hypertensive encephalopathy: Clues to pathogenesis. AJNR. American Journal of Neuroradiology. 1998;**19**:859-862

[18] Trommer BL, Homer D, Mikhael MA. Cerebral vasospasm and eclampsia. Stroke. 1988;**19**:326-329. DOI: 10.1161/01.str.19.3.326

[19] Parasher A, Jhamb R. Posterior reversible encephalopathy syndrome (PRES): Presentation, diagnosis and treatment. Postgraduate Medical Journal. 2020;**96**:623-628. DOI: 10.1136/postgradmedj-2020-137706

[20] Sesar A, Cavar I, Sesar AP, Sesar I. Transient cortical blindness in posterior reversible encephalopathy syndrome after postpartum eclampsia. Taiwan Journal of Ophthalmology. 2018;**8**:111-114. DOI: 10.4103/tjo.tjo_5_18

[21] Hugonneta E, Inesa DD, Boby H, Claise B, Petitcolin V, Lannareix V, et al. Posterior reversible encephalopathy syndrome (PRES): Features on CT and MR imaging. Diagnostic and Interventional Imaging. 2013;**94**:45-52. DOI: 10.1016/j.diii.2012.02.005

[22] Roth C, Ferbert A. Posterior reversible encephalopathy syndrome: Long-term follow-up. Journal of Neurology, Neurosurgery, and Psychiatry. 2010;**81**:773-777. DOI: 10.1136/jnnp.2009.189647

[23] Garg RK, Kumar N, Malhotra HS. Posterior reversible encephalopathy syndrome in eclampsia. Neurology India. 2018;**66**:1316-1323. DOI: 10.4103/0028-3886.241364

[24] Singh K, Jain D, Wallang B. Purtscher's retinopathy in pre-eclampsia: A blinding combination. International Ophthalmology. 2014;**34**:103-106. DOI: 10.1007/s10792-013-9739-1

[25] Tung CF, Peng YC, Chen GH, Chow WK, Yang DY, Hu WH. Hemolysis, elevated liver enzymes, and low platelet count (HELLP) syndrome with acute cortical blindness. Zhonghua Yi Xue Za Zhi (Taipei). 2001; **64**:482-485

[26] Mourelo M, Alvarez M, Díaz JL, García T, Galeiras R, Freire D. Postpartum amaurosis in a woman with severe preeclampsia. Indian Journal of Critical Care Medicine. 2011;**15**:227-229. DOI: 10.4103/0972-5229.92077

[27] Abu SK. The eye and visual system in the preeclampsia/eclampsia syndrome: What to expect? Saudi Journal of Ophthalmology. 2013;**27**:51-53. DOI: 10.1016/j.sjopt.2012.04.003

[28] Servillo G, Striano P, Striano S, Tortora F, Boccella P, De Robertis E, et al. Posterior reversible encephalopathy syndrome (PRES) in critically ill obstetric patients. Intensive Care Medicine. 2003;**29**:2323-2326. DOI: 10.1007/s00134-003-1901-1

[29] Hauswald M. Cortical blindness and late postpartum eclampsia. The American Journal of Emergency Medicine. 1987;**5**:130-132. DOI: 10.1016/0735-6757(87)90091-x

[30] Cunningham FG, Fernandez CO, Hernandez C. Blindness associated with preeclampsia and eclampsia. American Journal of Obstetrics and Gynecology. 1995;**172**:1291-1298. DOI: 10.1016/0002-9378(95)91495-1

[31] Roos NM, Wiegman MJ, Jansonius NM, Zeeman GG. Visual disturbances in (pre)eclampsia. Obstetrical & Gynecological Survey. 2012;**67**:242-250. DOI: 10.1097/OGX.0b013e318250a457

[32] Delefosse D, Samain E, Helias A, Regimbeau JM, Deval B, Farah E, et al. Late onset of cortical blindness in a patient with severe preeclampsia related to retained placental fragments. Anesthesiology. 2003;**98**:261-263. DOI: 10.1097/00000542-200301000-00038

[33] Wilson SJ, Best RM, Love M, Kamel H. Cortical blindness following pre-eclampsia. Eye (London, England). 2000;**14**:254-256. DOI: 10.1038/eye.2000.70

[34] Torres PJ, Antolin E, Gratacós E, Chamorro A, Cararach V. Cortical blindness in preeclampsia: Diagnostic evaluation by transcranial Doppler and magnetic resonance imaging techniques. Acta Obstetricia et Gynecologica Scandinavica. 1995;**74**:642-644. DOI: 10.3109/00016349509013479

[35] Llovera I, Roit Z, Johnson A, Sherman L. Cortical blindness, a rare complication of pre-eclampsia. The Journal of Emergency Medicine. 2005;**29**:295-297. DOI: 10.1016/j.jemermed.2005.03.008

[36] Borromeo CJ, Blike GT, Wiley CW, Hirsch JA. Cortical blindness in a preeclamptic patient after a cesarean delivery complicated by hypotension. Anesthesia and Analgesia. 2000;**91**:609-611. DOI: 10.1097/00000539-200009000-00021

[37] Rasdi AR, Nik-Ahmad-Zuky NL, Bakiah S, Shatriah I. Hypertensive retinopathy and visual outcome in hypertensive disorders in pregnancy. The Medical Journal of Malaysia. 2011;**66**:42-47

[38] Reddy SC, Nalliah S, George SRA, Who TS. Fundus changes in pregnancy induced hypertension. International Journal of Ophthalmology. 2012;**5**:694-697. DOI: 10.3980/j.issn.2222-3959.2012.06.08

[39] Rodríguez NA, Zurutuza A. Manifestaciones oftalmológicas de la hipertensión arterial [ophthalmological manifestations of arterial hypertension]. Anales del Sistema Sanitario de Navarra. 2008;**31**:13-22

[40] Prado RS, Figueiredo EL, Magalhães TVB. Retinal detachment in preeclampsia. Arquivos Brasileiros de Cardiologia. 2002;**79**:183-186. DOI: 10.1590/s0066-782x2002001100011

[41] Sunness JS. The pregnant women's eye. Surv Ophthalmol. Vol. 32; 1988. p. 219-238

[42] Katsimpris JM, Theoulakis PE, Manolopoulou P, Brinkmann CK, Gatzogias MI, Petropoulos IK. Bilateral serous retinal detachment in a case of preeclampsia. Klinische Monatsblätter für Augenheilkunde. 2009;**226**:352-354. DOI: 10.1055/s-0028-1109252

[43] Younis MT, McKibbin M, Wright A. Bilateral exudative retinal detachment causing blindness in severe pre-eclampsia. Journal of Obstetrics and Gynaecology. 2007;**27**:847-848. DOI: 10.1080/01443610701803891

[44] Blodi BA, Johnson MW, Gass JD, Fine SL, Joffe LM. Purtscher's-like retinopathy after childbirth. Ophthalmology. 1990;**97**:1654-1659. DOI: 10.1016/s0161-6420(90)32365-5

[45] Lara-Torre E, Lee MS, Wolf MA, Dinesh MS. Bilateral retinal occlusion progressing to long-lasting blindness in severe preeclampsia. Obstetrics and Gynecology. 2002;**100**:940-942. DOI: 10.1016/S0029-7844(02)02181-6

[46] Stewart MW, Brazis PW, Guier CP, Thota SH, Wilson SD. Purtscher-like retinopathy in a patient with HELLP

syndrome. American Journal of Ophthalmology. 2007;**143**:886-887. DOI: 10.1016/j.ajo.2006.12.005

[47] Agrawal A, McKibbin MA. Purtscher's and Purtscher-like retinopathies: A review. Survey of Ophthalmology. 2006;**51**:129-136. DOI: 10.1016/j.survophthal.2005.12.003

[48] Giridhar P, Freedman K. Nonarteritic anterior ischemic optic neuropathy in a 35-year-old postpartum woman with recent preeclampsia. JAMA Ophthalmology. 2013;**131**:542-544. DOI: 10.1001/jamaophthalmol.2013.2884

[49] Beck RW, Gamel JW, Willcourt RJ, Berman G. Acute ischemic optic neuropathy in severe preeclampsia. American Journal of Ophthalmology. 1980;**90**:342-346. DOI: 10.1016/s0002-9394(14)74914-1

[50] Ehlers JP, Fekret S. Retinal vein occlusion: Beyond the acute event. Survey of Ophthalmology. 2011;**56**:281-299. DOI: 0.1016/j.survophthal.2010.11.006

[51] Rahman I, Saleemi G, Semple D, Stanga P. Pre-eclampsia resulting in central retinal vein occlusion. Eye (London, England). 2006;**20**:955-957. DOI: 10.1038/sj.eye.6702065

[52] Kirfan G, Arunachalam M. Bilateral central retinal artery occlusion in pregnant women with severe preeclampsia post caesarian section delivery. American Journal of Respiratory and Critical Care Medicine. 2016;**193**:A6931

[53] Shilpa YD, Kalpana BN, Sheetal. Bilateral central retinal artery occlusion in a case of eclampsia. Egypt Retina Journal. 2018;**2**:50-52. DOI: 10.4103/erj.erj_8_18

[54] Capoor S, Goble RR, Wheatley T, Casswell AG. White-centered retinal hemorrhages as an early sign of preeclampsia. American Journal of Ophthalmology. 1995;**119**:804-806. DOI: 10.1016/s0002-9394(14)72793-x

[55] Leff SR, Yarian DL, Masciulli L, Green SN, Baldomero RE. Vitreous haemorrhage as a complication of HELLP syndrome. The British Journal of Ophthalmology. 1990;**74**:498. DOI: 10.1136/bjo.74.8.498